Lecture Notes:
Ophthalmology

We dedicate this book to Chris Chew, co-contributor and our esteemed friend and colleague, who died in 2004. We valued his insightful contributions, and his company is missed.

Lecture Notes
Ophthalmology

Bruce James
MA, DM, FRCS (Ed), FRCOphth
Consultant Ophthalmologist
Department of Ophthalmology
Stoke Mandeville Hospital
Buckinghamshire

Chris Chew
FRCS (Glasg), FRCOphth
Consultant Ophthalmologist
Late of Wolverhampton and Midland Counties Eye Infirmary
Wolverhampton

Anthony Bron
BSc, FRCS, FRCOphth, FMedSci
Professor of Ophthalmology
Nuffield Laboratory of Ophthalmology
Oxford

Tenth Edition

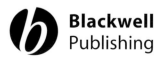

Blackwell
Publishing

First published 1960   Sixth edition 1980
Second edition 1965   Seventh edition 1986
Third edition 1968   Eighth edition 1997
Fourth edition 1971   Ninth edition 2003
Fifth edition 1974   Tenth edition 2007

1   2007

ISBN: 978-1-4051-5709-4

Catalogue records for this title are available from the British Library and the Library of
Congress

Set in 8/12pt Stone Serif by Graphicraft Limited, Hong Kong
Printed and bound in Singapore by COS Printers Pte Ltd

Commissioning Editor: Vicki Noyes
Editorial Assistant: Robin Harries
Development Editor: Beckie Brand
Production Controller: Debbie Wyer

For further information on Blackwell Publishing, visit our website:
http://www.blackwellpublishing.com

The publisher's policy is to use permanent paper from mills that operate a sustainable
forestry policy, and which has been manufactured from pulp processed using acid-free and
elementary chlorine-free practices. Furthermore, the publisher ensures that the text paper
and cover board used have met acceptable environmental accreditation standards.

Contents

Preface to tenth edition

If you are a student, just starting ophthalmology, you are probably already stretched by a busy curriculum. Suddenly you are asked to absorb an unfamiliar anatomy, new diseases and a fresh terminology. *Lecture Notes: Ophthalmology* aims to make this a palatable process.

Fortunately the discipline has many attractive features. Technologically, optical and digital techniques give diagnostic access to the minute structures of the eye. Specular microscopy can image the corneal endothelial cells which regulate corneal hydration and transparency; digital fluorescein angiography allows the retinal capillary bed to be explored in ischaemic retinal disease; optical coherence tomography allows the layers of the retina to be dissected and confocal microscopy provides a three-dimensional view of the optic nerve head. The shape of the cornea can be plotted digitally and, outside the globe, orbital structures and the visual pathway can be viewed by neuroimaging. Therapeutically, lasers are used to treat an extraordinary range of disorders, for instance, to break the cycle of events which cause angle closure glaucoma, to bring down pressure in chronic glaucoma, to open up an opaque lens capsule following cataract surgery, and to seal retinal holes. Sight-threatening diabetic retinopathy can be treated effectively by retinal photocoagulation, which ablates the ischaemic retina and removes the angiogenic stimulus to vasoproliferation. New treatments for macular degeneration, a major cause of visual disability in the Western world, are also showing promise.

The opportunities afforded by these techniques are matched by significant technological innovations in microsurgery, responsible for dramatic advances in cataract and vitreoretinal surgery. Cataracts are now removed by phacoemulsification, using an oscillating ultrasonic probe, and optical function is restored by insertion of a lens which unfolds within the eye. Vitreoretinal surgery employs inert gases to flatten the detached retina and endoscopic probes which allow manipulations in the vitreous space and the dissection of microscopic membranes from the retinal surface. Despite these advance most ophthalmic diagnoses can be made from a good history and clinical examination of the eye.

This book aims to give you skills which will be useful, whatever your final goal in medicine. Many systemic disorders have ocular features, and they may be critical in diagnosis. You will do well to learn the ophthalmic features of systemic hypertension, diabetes, sarcoidosis, endocarditis, demyelinating disease and space-occupying lesions of the brain, learn to recognize iritis and distinguish various forms of retinopathy and the difference between papilloedema and papillitis. This book will give you some help in this.

This tenth edition of *Lecture Notes: Ophthalmology* is very different from its predecessors. Each chapter starts with a set of learning objectives, and key points are summarized at the end of the clinical chapters. Bullet lists are used freely for emphasis. Test your understanding with the multiple choice and picture quiz questions at the end of each chapter. A new chapter on tropical ophthalmology is included, and the anatomical description of eye disease is complemented by a chapter on presenting symptoms. The final chapter offers 20 classical case histories, which will let you test your diagnostic skills. The final section of the book provides a list of further reading and the details of attractive websites which offer an expanded view of the specialty. Try some of these out.

We hope that you have as much fun reading these Lecture Notes as we did putting it all together.

Bruce James
Anthony Bron

Preface to first edition

This little guide does not presume to tell the medical student all that he needs to know about ophthalmology, for there are many larger books that do. But the medical curriculum becomes yearly more congested, while ophthalmology, still the 'Cinderella' of medicine, is generally left until the last, and only too readily goes by default. So it is to these harassed final-year students that the book is principally offered, in the sincere hope that they will find it useful; for nearly all eye diseases are recognized quite simply by their appearance, and a guide to ophthalmology need be little more than a gallery of pictures, linked by lecture notes.

My second excuse for publishing these lecture notes is a desire I have always had to escape from the traditional textbook presentation of ophthalmology as a string of small isolated diseases, with long unfamiliar names, and a host of eponyms. To the nineteenth-century empiricist, it seemed proper to classify a long succession of ocular structures, all of which emerged as isolated brackets for yet another sub-catalogue of small and equally isolated diseases. Surely it is time now to try and harness these miscellaneous ailments, not in terms of their diverse morphology, but in simpler clinical patterns; not as the microscopist lists them, but in the different ways that eye diseases present. For this, after all, is how the student will soon be meeting them.

I am well aware of the many inadequacies and omissions in this form of presentation, but if the belaboured student finds these lecture notes at least more readable, and therefore more memorable, than the prolix and time-honoured pattern, perhaps I will be justified.

Patrick Trevor-Roper

Acknowledgements

Numerous colleagues have provided valuable advice in their specialist areas, for which we are most grateful. The authors wish to thank Ramona Khooshabeh, Richard Smith, Larry Benjamin and Consuela Moorman for providing additional pictures for the tenth edition. We are particularly grateful to Professor Allen Foster at the London School of Hygiene and Tropical Medicine, who kindly provided the illustrations for the chapter on tropical ophthalmology. Thanks are due also to our editors and the staff at Blackwell Publishing for their encouragement, efficiency and patience during the production of this edition. We are also grateful to our copy-editor, Hugh Brazier, for his meticulous reading of the text and useful contributions to the style of the book.

Bruce James
Anthony Bron

Chapter 1

Anatomy

Learning objectives

To learn the anatomy of the eye, orbit and the third, fourth and sixth cranial nerves, to permit an understanding of medical conditions affecting these structures.

Introduction

A knowledge of ocular anatomy and function is important to the understanding of eye diseases. A brief outline is given below.

Gross anatomy

The eye (Fig. 1.1) comprises:

- A tough outer coat which is transparent anteriorly (the *cornea*) and opaque posteriorly (the *sclera*). The junction between the two is called the *limbus*. The extraocular muscles attach to the outer sclera while the optic nerve leaves the globe posteriorly.
- A rich vascular coat (the *uvea*) forms the *choroid* posteriorly, which is lined by and firmly attached to the retina. The choroid nourishes the outer two-thirds of the retina. Anteriorly, the uvea forms the ciliary body and the iris.
- The *ciliary body* contains the smooth *ciliary muscle*, whose contraction allows lens shape to alter and the focus of the eye to be changed. The ciliary epithelium secretes *aqueous humour* and maintains the ocular pressure. The ciliary body provides attachment for the *iris*, which forms the pupillary diaphragm.

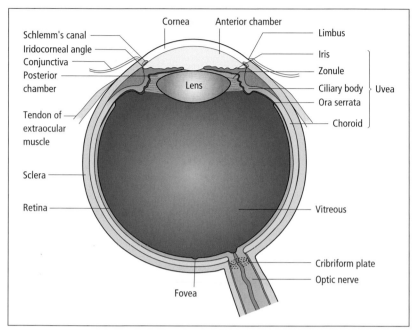

Figure 1.1 The basic anatomy of the eye.

- The *lens* lies behind the iris and is supported by fine fibrils (the *zonule*) running under tension between the lens and the ciliary body.
- The angle formed by the iris and cornea (the *iridocorneal angle*) is lined by a meshwork of cells and collagen beams (the *trabecular meshwork*). In the sclera outside this, *Schlemm's canal* conducts the aqueous humour from the anterior chamber into the venous system, permitting aqueous drainage. This region is thus also termed the *drainage angle*.

The cornea anteriorly and the iris and central lens posteriorly form the *anterior chamber*. Between the iris, the lens and the ciliary body lies the *posterior chamber* (distinct from the *vitreous body*). Both these chambers are filled with aqueous humour. Between the lens and the retina lies the vitreous body, occupying most of the posterior segment of the eye.

Anteriorly, the *bulbar conjunctiva* of the globe is reflected from the sclera onto the underside of the eyelids to form the *tarsal conjunctiva*. A connective tissue layer (*Tenon's capsule*) separates the conjunctiva from the sclera and is prolonged backwards as a sheath around the rectus muscles.

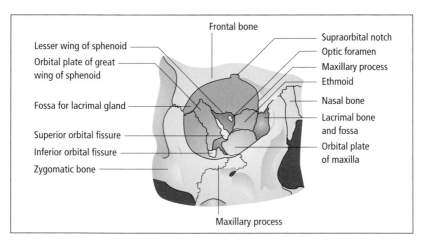

Figure 1.2 The anatomy of the orbit.

The orbit

The eye lies within the bony orbit, which has the shape of a four-sided pyramid (Fig. 1.2). At its posterior apex is the *optic canal*, which transmits the optic nerve to the chiasm, tract and lateral geniculate body. The *superior and inferior orbital fissures* allow the passage of blood vessels and cranial nerves which supply orbital structures. The *lacrimal gland* lies anteriorly in the superolateral aspect of the orbit. On the anterior medial wall lies the fossa for the *lacrimal sac*.

The eyelids (tarsal plates)

The eyelids (Fig. 1.3):
- offer mechanical protection to the anterior globe;
- spread the tear film over the conjunctiva and cornea with each blink;
- contain the *meibomian oil glands*, which provide the lipid component of the tear film;
- prevent drying of the eyes;
- contain the puncta through which the tears flow into the lacrimal drainage system.
They comprise:
- an anterior layer of skin;
- the *orbicularis muscle*, whose contraction results in forced eye closure;
- a tough collagenous layer (the *tarsal plate*) which houses the oil glands;
- an epithelial lining, the tarsal conjunctiva, which is reflected onto the globe via the *fornices*.

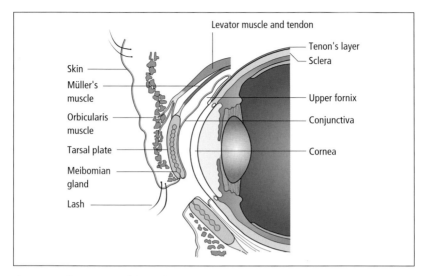

Figure 1.3 The anatomy of the eyelids.

The *levator muscle* passes forwards to the upper lid and inserts into the tarsal plate. It is innervated by the third nerve. Damage to the nerve or lid changes in old age result in drooping of the eyelid (*ptosis*). A flat smooth muscle arising from the deep surface of the levator inserts into the tarsal plate. It is innervated by the sympathetic nervous system. If the sympathetic supply is damaged (as in Horner's syndrome) a slight ptosis results.

The meibomian oil glands deliver their oil to the skin of the lid margin, just anterior to the *mucocutaneous junction*. This oil is layered onto the anterior surface of the tear film with each blink, where it retards evaporation. Far medially on the lid margins, two puncta form the initial part of the lacrimal drainage system.

The lacrimal drainage system

Tears drain into the upper and lower *puncta* and then into the *lacrimal sac* via the upper and lower *canaliculi* (Fig. 1.4). They form a common canaliculus before entering the lacrimal sac. The *nasolacrimal duct* passes from the sac to the nose. Failure of the distal part of the nasolacrimal duct to fully canalize at birth is the usual cause of a watering, sticky eye in a baby. Tear drainage is an active process. Each blink of the lids helps to pump tears through the system.

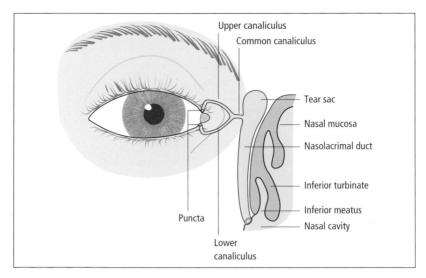

Figure 1.4 The major components of the lacrimal drainage system

Detailed functional anatomy

The tear film

The ocular surface is bathed constantly by the tears, secreted mainly by the lacrimal gland but supplemented by conjunctival secretions. They drain away via the nasolacrimal system.

The ocular surface cells express a mucin *glycocalyx* which renders the surface wettable. When the eyes are open, the exposed ocular surface (the cornea and nasal and temporal wedges of conjunctiva) are covered by a thin tear film, 3 μm thick, which comprises three layers:

1 a thin *mucin layer* in contact with the ocular surface and produced mainly by the conjunctival goblet cells;

2 an *aqueous layer* produced by the lacrimal gland;

3 a surface *oil layer* produced by the tarsal meibomian glands and delivered to the lid margins.

Functions of the tear film

● It provides a smooth air/tear interface for distortion-free refraction of light at the cornea.

● It provides oxygen anteriorly to the avascular cornea.

• It removes debris and foreign particles from the ocular surface through the flow of tears.
• It has antibacterial properties through the action of lysozyme, lactoferrin, defensins and the immunoglobulins, particularly secretory IgA.
The tear film is replenished with each blink.

The cornea

The cornea (Fig. 1.5) is 0.5 mm thick and comprises:
• The *epithelium*, an anterior non-keratinized squamous layer, thickened peripherally at the *limbus* where it is continuous with the conjunctiva. The limbus houses the germinative *stem cells* of the corneal epithelium.
• An underlying *stroma* of collagen fibrils, ground substance and fibroblasts. The regular packing, small diameter and narrow separation of the collagen fibrils account for corneal transparency. This orderly architecture is maintained by regulating stromal hydration.
• The *endothelium*, a monolayer of non-regenerating cells which actively pump ions and water from the stroma, controlling corneal hydration and hence transparency. The difference between the regenerative capacity of the epithelium and endothelium is important. Damage to the epithelial layer, by an abrasion for example, is rapidly repaired by cell spreading and proliferation. Endothelial damage, by disease or surgery, is repaired by cell spreading alone, with a loss of cell density. A point is reached when loss of its barrier and pumping functions leads to overhydration (oedema), disruption of the regular packing of its stromal collagen and corneal clouding.

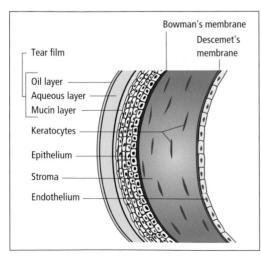

Figure 1.5 The structure of the cornea and precorneal tear film (schematic, not to scale – the stroma accounts for 95% of the corneal thickness).

The nutrition of the cornea is supplied almost entirely by the aqueous humour, which circulates through the anterior chamber and bathes the posterior surface of the cornea. The aqueous also supplies oxygen to the posterior stroma, while the anterior stroma receives its oxygen from the ambient air. The oxygen supply to the anterior cornea is reduced but still sufficient during lid closure, but a too-tightly fitting contact lens may deprive the anterior cornea of oxygen and cause corneal, especially epithelial, oedema.

Functions of the cornea
• It protects the internal ocular structures.
• Together with the lens, it refracts and focuses light onto the retina. The junction between the ambient air and the curved surface of the cornea, covered by its optically smooth tear film, forms a powerful refractive interface.

The sclera

• The sclera is formed from interwoven collagen fibrils of different widths lying within a ground substance and maintained by fibroblasts.
• It is of variable thickness, 1 mm around the optic nerve head and 0.3 mm just posterior to the muscle insertions.

The choroid

• The choroid (Fig. 1.6) is formed of arterioles, venules and a dense fenestrated capillary network.
• It is loosely attached to the sclera.
• It has a remarkably high blood flow.
• It nourishes the deep, outer layers of the retina and may have a role in its temperature homeostasis.
• Its basement membrane, together with that of the retinal pigment epithelium (RPE), forms the acellular Bruch's membrane, which acts as a diffusion barrier between the choroid and the retina.

The retina

The retina (Fig. 1.7) is a highly complex structure derived embryologically from the primitive optic cup.

Its outermost layer is the retinal pigment epithelium (RPE) while its innermost layer forms the neuroretina, consisting of the photoreceptors (*rods* and *cones*), the bipolar nerve layer (and additional nerve cells) and the *ganglion cell* layer, whose axons give rise to the innermost, nerve fibre layer. These nerve fibres converge to the optic nervehead, where they form the optic nerve.

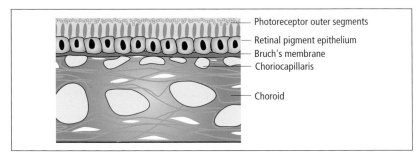

Figure 1.6 The relationship between the choroid, RPE and retina.

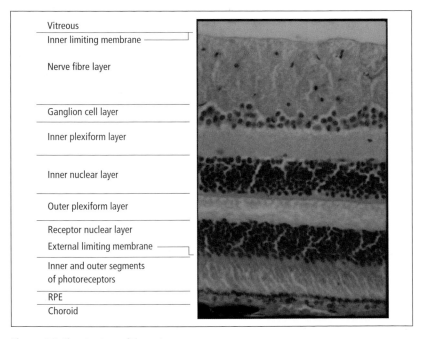

Figure 1.7 The structure of the retina.

The retinal pigment epithelium (RPE)

- is formed from a single layer of cells;
- is loosely attached to the neuro retina except at the periphery (*ora serrata*) and around the optic disc;

- forms microvilli which project between and embrace the outer segment discs of the rods and cones;
- phagocytoses the redundant external segments of the rods and cones;
- facilitates the passage of nutrients and metabolites between the retina and choroid;
- takes part in the regeneration of rhodopsin and cone opsin, the photoreceptor visual pigments and in recycling vitamin A;
- contains melanin granules which absorb light scattered by the sclera thereby enhancing image formation on the retina.

The photoreceptor layer

The photoreceptor layer is responsible for converting light into electrical signals. The initial integration of these signals is also performed by the retina.
- *Cones* (Fig. 1.8) are responsible for daylight and colour vision and have a relatively high threshold to light. Different subgroups of cones are responsive to short, medium and long wavelengths (blue, green, red). They are concentrated at the fovea, which is responsible for detailed vision such as reading fine print.
- *Rods* are responsible for night vision. They have a low light threshold and do not signal wavelength information (colour). They form the large majority of photoreceptors in the remaining retina.

The vitreous

- The vitreous is a clear gel occupying two-thirds of the globe.
- It is 98% water. The remainder is gel-forming hyaluronic acid traversed by a fine collagen network. There are few cells.
- It is firmly attached anteriorly to the peripheral retina, *pars plana* and around the optic disc, and less firmly to the macula and retinal vessels.
- It has a nutritive and supportive role.

Collapse of the vitreous gel (vitreous detachment), which is common in later life, puts traction on points of attachment and may occasionally lead to a peripheral retinal break or hole, where the vitreous pulls off a flap of the underlying retina.

The ciliary body

The ciliary body (Fig. 1.9) is subdivided into three parts:
1 the *ciliary muscle*;
2 the ciliary processes (*pars plicata*);
3 the *pars plana*.

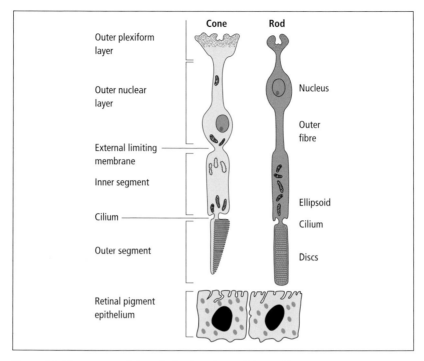

Figure 1.8 The structure of the retinal rods and cones (schematic).

The ciliary muscle
- This comprises smooth muscle arranged in a ring overlying the ciliary processes.
- It is innervated by the parasympathetic system via the third cranial nerve.
- It is responsible for changes in lens thickness and curvature during *accommodation*. The *zonular fibres* supporting the lens are under tension during distant viewing, giving the lens a flattened profile. Contraction of the muscle *relaxes* the zonule and permits the elasticity of the lens to *increase* its curvature and hence its refractive power.

The ciliary processes (pars plicata)
- There are about 70 radial *ciliary processes* arranged in a ring around the posterior chamber. They are responsible for the secretion of aqueous humour.
- Each ciliary process is formed by an epithelium two layers thick (the outer *pigmented* and the inner *non-pigmented*) with a vascular stroma.
- The stromal capillaries are fenestrated, allowing plasma constituents ready access.

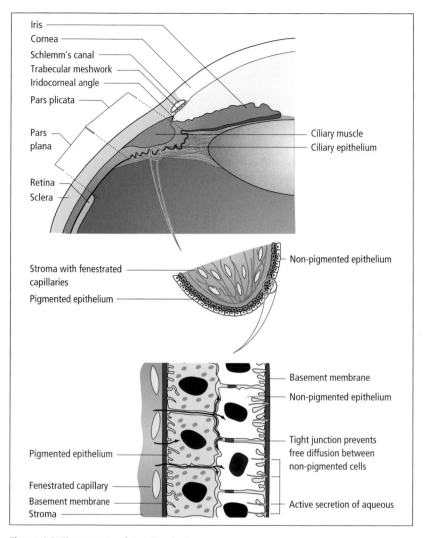

Figure 1.9 The anatomy of the ciliary body.

● The *tight junctions* between the non-pigmented epithelial cells provide a barrier to free diffusion into the posterior chamber. They are essential for the active secretion of aqueous by the non-pigmented cells.
● The epithelial cells show marked infolding, which significantly increases their surface area for fluid and solute transport.

The pars plana
- This comprises a relatively avascular stroma covered by an epithelial layer two cells thick.
- It is safe to make surgical incisions through the scleral wall here to gain access to the vitreous cavity.

The iris

- The iris is attached peripherally to the anterior part of the ciliary body.
- It forms the *pupil* at its centre, the aperture of which can be varied by the circular *sphincter* and radial *dilator* muscles to control the amount of light entering the eye.
- It has an anterior border layer of fibroblasts and collagen and a cellular stroma in which the sphincter muscle is embedded at the pupil margin.
- The sphincter muscle is innervated by the *parasympathetic* system.
- The smooth dilator muscle extends from the iris periphery towards the sphincter. It is innervated by the *sympathetic* system.
- Posteriorly the iris is lined by a pigmented epithelium two layers thick.

The iridocorneal (drainage) angle

This lies between the iris, the anterior tip of the ciliary body and the cornea. It is the site of aqueous drainage from the eye via the trabecular meshwork (Fig. 1.10).

The trabecular meshwork

This overlies Schlemm's canal and is composed of a lattice of collagen beams covered by trabecular cells. The spaces between these beams become increasingly small as Schlemm's canal is approached. The outermost zone of the meshwork accounts for most of the resistance to aqueous outflow. Damage here raises the resistance and increases intraocular pressure in primary open angle glaucoma. Some of the spaces may be blocked and there is a reduction in the number of cells covering the trabecular beams (see Chapter 10).

Fluid passes into Schlemm's canal both through giant vacuoles in its endothelial lining and through intercellular spaces.

The lens

The lens (Fig. 1.11) is the second major refractive element of the eye; the cornea, with its tear film, is the first.

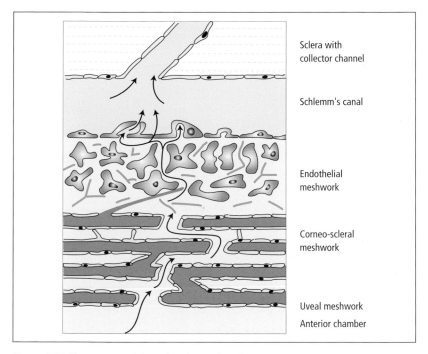

Sclera with
collector channel

Schlemm's canal

Endothelial
meshwork

Corneo-scleral
meshwork

Uveal meshwork

Anterior chamber

Figure 1.10 The anatomy of the trabecular meshwork.

- It grows throughout life.
- It is supported by zonular fibres running between the ciliary body and the lens capsule.
- It comprises an outer collagenous capsule under whose anterior part lies a monolayer of epithelial cells. Towards the *equator* the epithelium gives rise to the lens fibres.
- The zonular fibres transmit changes in the ciliary muscle, allowing the lens to change its shape and refractive power.
- The lens fibres make up the bulk of the lens. They are elongated cells arranged in layers which arch over the lens equator. Anteriorly and posteriorly they meet to form the lens *sutures*. With age the deeper *fibres* lose their nuclei and intracellular organelles.
- The oldest central fibres represent the fetal lens and form the lens *nucleus*; the peripheral fibres make up the lens *cortex*.
- The high refractive index of the lens arises from the high protein content of its fibres.

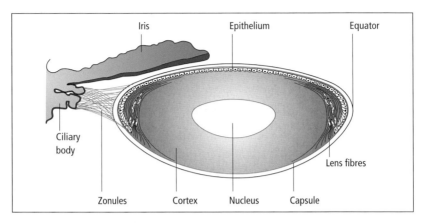

Figure 1.11 The anatomy of the lens.

The optic nerve

• The optic nerve (Fig. 1.12) is formed by the axons arising from the *retinal ganglion cell layer*, which form the *nerve fibre layer* of the retina.

• It passes out of the eye through the cribriform plate of the sclera, a sieve-like structure.

• In the orbit the optic nerve is surrounded by a sheath formed by the dura, arachnoid and pia mater, continuous with that surrounding the brain. It is bathed in cerebrospinal fluid.

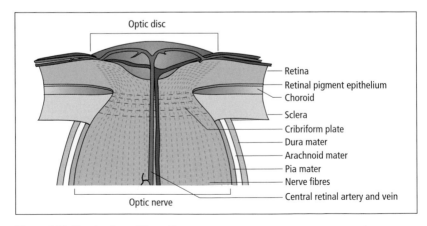

Figure 1.12 The structure of the optic nerve.

The central retinal artery and vein enter the eye in the centre of the optic nerve. The extraocular nerve fibres are myelinated; those within the eye are not.

The ocular blood supply

The eye receives its blood supply from the ophthalmic artery (a branch of the internal carotid artery) via the retinal artery, ciliary arteries and muscular arteries (Fig. 1.13). The conjunctival circulation anastomoses anteriorly with branches from the external carotid artery.

The anterior optic nerve is supplied by branches from the ciliary arteries. The inner retina is supplied by arterioles branching from the central retinal artery. These arterioles each supply an area of retina, with little overlap. Obstruction results in ischaemia of most of the area supplied by that arteriole. The fovea is so thin that it requires no supply from the retinal circulation. It is supplied indirectly, as are the outer layers of the retina, by diffusion of oxygen and metabolites across the retinal pigment epithelium from the choroid.

The endothelial cells of the retinal capillaries are joined by tight junctions so that the vessels are impermeable to proteins. This forms an '*inner blood retinal barrier*', with properties similar to that of the blood–brain barrier. The capillaries of the choroid, however, are fenestrated and leaky. The retinal pigment epithelial cells are also joined by tight junctions and present an '*external blood–retinal barrier*' between the leaky choroid and the retina.

The breakdown of these barriers causes the retinal signs seen in many vascular diseases.

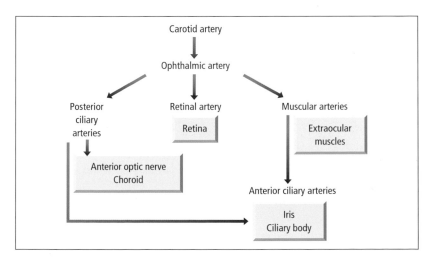

Figure 1.13 Diagrammatic representation of the ocular blood supply.

Table 1.1 The muscles and tissues supplied by the third, fourth and sixth cranial nerves.

Third (oculomotor)	Fourth (trochlear)	Sixth (abducens)
Medial rectus	Superior oblique	Lateral rectus
Inferior rectus		
Superior rectus (innervated by the contralateral nucleus)		
Inferior oblique		
Levator palpebrae (both levators are innervated by a single midline nucleus)		
Preganglionic parasympathetic fibres end in the ciliary ganglion. Here postganglionic fibres arise and pass in the short ciliary nerves to the sphincter pupillae and the ciliary muscle		

The third, fourth and sixth cranial nerves

The structures supplied by each of these nerves are shown in Table 1.1.

Central origin

The nuclei of the third (oculomotor) and fourth (trochlear) cranial nerves lie in the midbrain; the sixth nerve (abducens) nuclei lie in the pons. Figure 1.14 shows some of the important relations of these nuclei and their fascicles.

Nuclear and fascicular palsies of these nerves are unusual. If they do occur they are associated with other neurological problems. For example if the third nerve fascicles are damaged as they pass through the red nucleus the ipsilateral third nerve palsy will be accompanied by a contralateral tremor. Furthermore a nuclear third nerve lesion results in a *contralateral* palsy of the superior rectus as the fibres from the subnucleus supplying this muscle cross.

Peripheral course

Figure 1.15 shows the intracranial course of the third, fourth and sixth cranial nerves.

Third nerve

The third nerve leaves the midbrain ventrally between the cerebral peduncles. It then passes between the *posterior cerebral* and *superior cerebellar arteries* and then

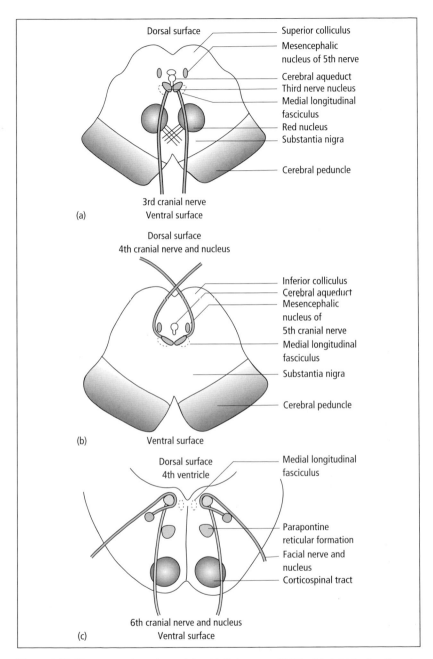

Figure 1.14 Diagrams to show the nuclei and initial course of (a) the third, (b) the fourth and (c) the sixth cranial nerves.

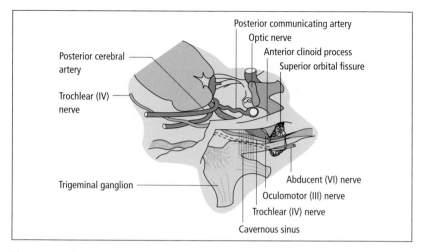

Figure 1.15 The intracranial course of the third, fourth and sixth cranial nerves.

lateral to the *posterior communicating artery*. Aneurysms of this artery may cause a third nerve palsy. The nerve enters the cavernous sinus in its lateral wall and enters the orbit through the superior orbital fissure.

Fourth nerve

The nerve decussates and leaves the *dorsal* aspect of the midbrain below the inferior colliculus. It first curves around the midbrain before passing like the third nerve between the posterior cerebral and superior cerebellar arteries to enter the lateral aspect of the cavernous sinus inferior to the third nerve. It enters the orbit via the superior orbital fissure.

Sixth nerve

Fibres leave from the inferior border of the pons. It has a long intracranial course passing upwards along the pons to angle anteriorly over the petrous bone and into the cavernous sinus where it lies infero-medial to the fourth nerve in proximity to the internal carotid artery. It enters the orbit through the superior orbital fissure. This long course is important because the nerve can be involved in numerous intracranial pathologies including base of skull fractures, invasion by nasopharyngeal tumours and raised intracranial pressure.

Multiple choice questions

1. The cornea

a Has an endothelial layer that regenerates readily.
b Comprises three layers.
c The endothelium actively pumps water from the stroma.
d Is an important refractive component of the eye.
e Has a stroma composed of randomly arranged collagen fibrils.

2. The retina

a Is ten layers thick.
b Has ganglion cells whose axons form the optic nerve.
c Has three types of rods responsible for colour vision.
d The neuroretina is firmly attached to the retinal pigment epithelium.
e The RPE delivers vitamin A for rhodopsin production.

3. The lens

a Grows throughout life.
b Is surrounded by a collagenous capsule.
c Cortical and nuclear fibres are nucleated.
d Has a high refractive index owing to its protein content.
e Changes in shape with accommodation.

4. The suspensory ligament of the lens (the zonule)

a Attaches the lens to the ciliary body.
b Is part of the iridocorneal angle.
c Is composed of smooth muscle.
d Transmits changes in tension to the lens capsule.

5. The posterior chamber

a Is another name for the vitreous body.
b Lies between the iris, lens and ciliary body.
c Contains aqueous humour, secreted by the ciliary processes.
d Is in communication with the anterior chamber.

6. The tear film

a Is 100 μm thick.
b Is composed of four layers.
c The mucin layer is in contact with the cornea.
d Is important in the refraction of light entering the eye.
e Contains lysozyme and secretory IgA.

7. The iridocorneal angle

a Is the site of aqueous production.
b Lies between the cornea and the ciliary body.
c In primary open angle glaucoma there is a reduction in the number of cells covering the trabecular meshwork.
d Fluid passes through the trabecular meshwork to Schlemm's canal.

8. The optic nerve

a Axons leave the eyeball through the cribriform plate.
b Is not bathed in CSF until it enters the cranial cavity.
c Anteriorly is supplied by blood from the ciliary arteries.
d Axons are not myelinated in its retrobulbar part.
e Is formed by the nerve fibre layer of the retina.

9. The third, fourth and sixth cranial nerves

a All originate in the midbrain.
b A *nuclear* third nerve palsy will cause a contralateral palsy of the superior rectus.
c The fourth nerve supplies the lateral rectus.
d The sixth nerve has a long intracranial course.
e The third nerve may be affected by aneurysms of the posterior communicating artery.

Answers

1. The cornea

a False. The human endothelium does not regenerate; dead cells are replaced by the spreading of surviving cells.
b True. The cornea has epithelial, stromal and endothelial layers.

c True. The endothelial cells pump out ions and the water follows osmotically. Removal of water maintains corneal transparency.

d True. The cornea is a more powerful refractive element than the natural lens of the eye.

e False. The fine, equally spaced, stromal collagen fibrils are arranged in parallel and packed in an orderly manner. This is a requirement for transparency.

2. The retina

a True. See Fig. 1.7.

b True. The retinal ganglion cell axons form the retinal nerve fibre layer and exit the eye at the optic nerve head.

c False. The rods are responsible for night vision and three cone types are responsible for daylight and colour vision.

d False. The attachment is loose; the neuroretina separates in retinal detachment.

e True. Vitamin A is delivered by the RPE to the photoreceptors and combined with opsin.

3. The lens

a True.

b True. This is of great importance in cataract surgery.

c False. The older, deep cortical and nuclear fibres lose their nuclei and other organelles.

d True.

e True.

4. The suspensory ligament of the lens (the zonule)

a True. Zonular fibres extend from the pars plicata of the ciliary body to the lens equator.

b False. The zonule lies behind the iris and iridocorneal angle.

c False. The ciliary muscle contains smooth muscle, not the zonule.

d True. Contraction of the ciliary muscle relaxes the zonular fibres allowing the lens to increase its curvature and thus its refractive power (this is 'accommodation').

5. The posterior chamber

a False. The vitreous body is quite separate.

b True.

c True.

d True. Communication is via the pupil, in the gap between iris and lens at the pupil margin. If this gap is narrowed or closed, pressure in the posterior chamber pushes the iris forward and may close the angle (acute closed angle glaucoma).

6. The tear film

a False. The tear film is 3 μm thick.
b False. The tear film is composed of mucin, aqueous and oil layers.
c True.
d True. It provides a smooth interface for the refraction of light.
e True.

7. The iridocorneal angle

a False. It is the site of aqueous drainage.
b True.
c True.
d True. The process is active.

8. The optic nerve

a True.
b False. In the orbit, within its sheaths, the optic nerve is surrounded by sub-arachnoid CSF in continuity with that in the intracranial cavity.
c True. This is a most important blood supply for the anterior optic nerve.
d False. They are usually not myelinated *within* the eye.
e True. It is made up from retinal ganglion cell axons.

9. The third, fourth and sixth cranial nerves

a False. The nucleus of the sixth nerve lies in the pons.
b True. The superior rectus is innervated by the contralateral nucleus.
c False. It supplies the superior oblique.
d True. This makes the sixth nerve susceptible to trauma, which may cause lateral rectus palsy.
e True. It passes lateral to the artery.

Chapter 2

History and examination

Learning objectives

To be able to:
- Take and understand an ophthalmic history.
- Examine the function of the eye (acuity and visual field).
- Test pupillary reactions.
- Examine eye movements.
- Examine the structure of the eye.
- Understand the use of fluorescein.
- Use the ophthalmoscope.

Introduction

Ophthalmic diagnosis is heavily dependent on a good history and a thorough examination. The majority of ophthalmic diagnoses do not require additional tests. The sequence of history and examination is described below. It is imperative that hands are washed following each examination. If ocular infection is suspected then it may be necessary to disinfect the slit lamp and other hand-held equipment. Equipment making contact with the eye, e.g. a diagnostic contact lens, is disposable or routinely disinfected.

History

A good history must include details of:
• Ocular symptoms, time of onset, eye affected, and associated non-ocular symptoms.

- Past ocular history (e.g. poor vision in one eye since birth, recurrence of previous disease, particularly inflammatory).
- Past medical history (e.g. of *hypertension*, which may be associated with some vascular eye diseases such as central retinal vein occlusion, *diabetes*, which may cause retinopathy, and systemic *inflammatory* disease such as sarcoid, which may also cause ocular inflammation).
- Drug history, since some drugs such as isoniazid and chloroquine may be toxic to the eye.
- Family history (e.g. of ocular diseases known to be inherited, such as retinitis pigmentosa, or of disease where family history may be a risk factor, such as glaucoma).
- Presence of allergies.

Examination

Both structure and function of the eye are examined.

Two common ophthalmic symptoms and additional questions that should be asked	
Loss of vision	Sudden/gradual Painful/painless Transient/permanent Both eyes/single eye/part of field
Red eye	Watery/sticky Painful With visual loss Duration

Physiological testing of the eye

Visual acuity

Adults
Visual acuity (VA) tests the visual resolving power of the eye. The standard test is the Snellen chart, consisting of rows of letters (known as optotypes) of decreasing size (Fig. 2.1a). Each row is numbered with the distance in metres at which each letter width subtends 1 minute of arc at the eye. Acuity is recorded as the reading distance (e.g. 6 metres) over the row number of the smallest letter seen. If this is the 6 metre line, then VA is 6/6; if it is the 60 metre line, then VA is 6/60. Visual resolution is ten times greater at 6/6 than 6/60. Some countries use a different scale, using the foot as the unit of distance, and 20/20 on this scale equates to 6/6.

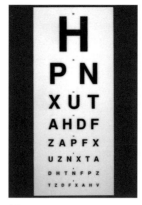

(a)

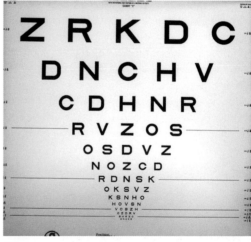

(b)

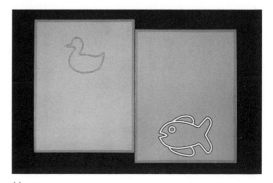

Figure 2.1 Methods of assessing visual acuity: (a) the Snellen chart; (b) a logMAR acuity chart; (c) examples of Cardiff cards.

(c)

Increasingly the logMAR visual acuity chart is being used, particularly in re-search (Fig. 2.1b). This standardizes the difference in letter size between each line. The number of letters on each line is equal, and the chart also allows accurate scor-ing of incompletely seen lines. Scores are recorded as a decimal, 0.00 equating to 6/6 (see Appendix).

Vision is tested with spectacles if worn, but viewing through a pinhole will cor-rect for moderate refractive error.

Children

In children, various methods are used to assess visual acuity:

• Very young children are observed to see if they can follow objects or pick up scattered 'hundreds and thousands' cake decorations.

• The Cardiff Acuity Test can be used to assess vision in one- to three-year-olds. This is a *preferential looking test* based on the finding that children prefer to look at complex rather than plain targets. The grey cards present a variety of figures sur-rounded by a white band bordered with two black bands (Fig. 2.1c). As the width of the bands decreases, the picture becomes harder to see against the grey back-ground. The gaze of the child is observed and the examiner estimates whether the object seen is at the top or bottom of the card. When the examiner is unable to identify the position of the object from the child's gaze it is assumed that the child cannot see the picture and the resolution of the eye is inferred.

• Older children are able to identify or match single pictures and letters of varying size (*Sheridan–Gardiner test*).

Visual fields

The visual fields map the peripheral extent of the visual world. Each field can be represented as a series of contours or *isoptres*, demonstrating the ability to resolve a target of given size and brightness at a particular location. The field is not flat; towards the centre the eye is able to detect much smaller objects than at the periphery. This produces a '*hill of vision*' in which objects which are resolved in finest detail are at the peak of the hill (at the *fovea*) and acuity falls towards the periphery (Fig. 2.2). On the temporal side of the field is the blind spot, which cor-responds to the position of the optic nerve head, where there are no photoreceptors.

The visual field may be tested in various ways.

Confrontation tests

One eye of the patient is covered and the examiner sits opposite, closing his eye on the same side. The test object, traditionally the head of a large hat pin, is then brought into view from the periphery and moved centrally. The patient is asked to say when he first sees the object. Each quadrant is tested and the location of the

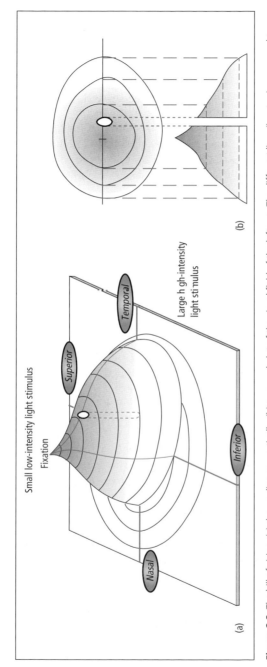

Figure 2.2 The hill of vision: (a) shown diagrammatically; (b) a normal plot of the visual field of the left eye. The different lines (isoptres) correspond to different sizes or intensities of the target. (Adapted with permission from Anderson, D.R. (1982) *Testing the Field of Vision*. Mosby-Year Book, Inc., St Louis.)

blind spot determined. The patient's field is thus compared with that of the examiner. With practice central *scotomas* can also be identified. (A scotoma is a focal area of decreased sensitivity within the field, surrounded by a more sensitive area.)

A crude test for hemianopic or quadrantic defects
- Sit facing the patient and hold your hands up, palms forwards, one on either side of the midline. Ask the patient to cover one eye and look directly at your face. Enquire if the two palms appear qualitatively the same. The patient may notice that the outer (temporal) palm appears duller. Repeat the test with the fellow eye. This can be useful in picking up a bitemporal hemianopia (patients may also miss the temporal letters on the Snellen chart when their visual acuity is measured).
- Ask the patient to count the number of fingers which you show in each quadrant of the visual field.

A useful test to identify a neurological field defect is to use a red object. The red field is the most sensitive to optic nerve lesions. A red-topped pin is used to perform a confrontation test, the patient being asked to say when he first sees the pin top as red (not when he first sees the pin top). More simply, a red object can be held in each quadrant or hemifield and the patient asked to compare the quality of red in each location. In a hemianopic field defect the red would appear duller in the affected field.

Perimeters
These machines permit more accurate plotting of the visual field. They measure:
- The *kinetic* visual field, in which the patient indicates when he first sees a light of a specific size and brightness brought in from the periphery. This is rather like the moving pinhead of the confrontation test.
- The *static* visual field, in which the patient indicates when he first sees the presentation of a stationary light of increasing brightness.

These techniques are particularly useful in chronic ocular and neurological conditions to monitor changes in the visual field (e.g. in glaucoma).

Increasingly sophisticated perimeters are being developed using computer programs that enable the time it takes to perform an accurate visual field to be reduced. These measure the threshold stimuli (the minimum intensity of light of a standard-sized source that the subject is able to see 50% of the time) for a number of points in the visual field. The intensity of light is recorded in decibels: the higher the number the dimmer the light (Fig. 2.3).

Perimeters that test different pathways in the visual system have also been developed. For example a flickering target tests the M-cell pathway, responsible for motion detection. These may be important in diseases that may selectively affect one pathway, such as glaucoma.

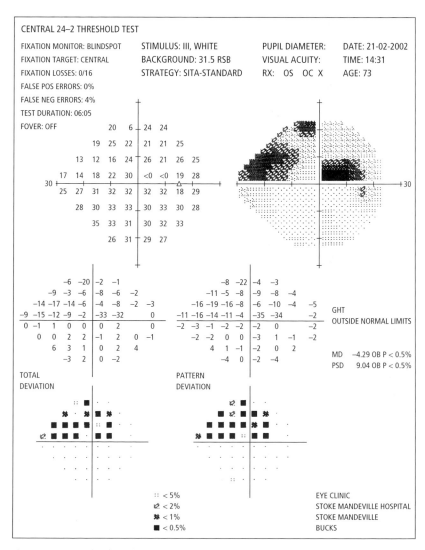

Figure 2.3 Example of a threshold field plot from an automated perimeter. The upper left diagram shows the threshold values for each test location. This is pictorially represented in the upper right picture. The middle diagrams compare the subject's field with that of a normal age-matched population. The lower diagrams indicate how likely it is that the value of each location differs from this control population.

Intraocular pressure

Intraocular pressure is measured by a contact technique, with a Goldmann tonometer (Fig. 2.4). A clear plastic cylinder is pressed against the anaesthetized cornea. The ring of flattening, viewed through the cylinder, is made visible by the presence of fluorescein in the tear film (see below). A horizontally disposed prism, within the cylinder, splits the ring of contact into two hemicircles. The force applied to the cylinder can be varied to alter the amount of corneal flattening and thus the size of the ring. It is adjusted so that the two hemicircles just interlock. This is the endpoint of the test and the force applied, converted into units of ocular pressure (mmHg), can now be read from the tonometer.

Optometrists use a puff of air of varying intensity to produce corneal flattening rather than the prism of the Goldmann tonometer. Various other tonometers are also available, including small hand-held electronic devices.

The thickness of the cornea has a significant effect on the measurement of intraocular pressure, affecting the accuracy of measurement with contact tonometers. These tonometers underestimate the pressure where the cornea is thin and easier to deform. A thicker cornea requires more force for the same deformation, leading to an overestimation of intraocular pressure. Measurement of corneal thickness can now readily be performed with small hand-held ultrasonic pachymeters, which are used increasingly to make the appropriate correction.

Pupillary reactions

The size of the pupils (*miosis*, constricted; *mydriasis*, dilated) and their response to light and accommodation give important information about:
• the function of the afferent pathway controlling the pupils (the optic nerve and tract) (see Chapter 13);
• the function of the efferent pathway;
• the action of drugs on the pupil.
Examination of the pupils begins with an assessment of the size and symmetry of the pupils in a uniform light. If there is asymmetry (*anisocoria*) it must be decided whether the small or large pupil is abnormal. A pathologically small pupil (after damage to the sympathetic nervous system) will be more apparent in dim illumination, since dilation of the normal pupil will be greater. A pathologically large pupil (seen in disease of the parasympathetic nervous system) will be more apparent in the light since the fellow pupil will be small.

While some individuals show pupil asymmetry unassociated with disease, remember that inflammation of the anterior segment (*iritis*), trauma or previous ocular surgery may cause structural iris changes which mechanically alter pupil shape or result in posterior synechiae (see Chapter 9).

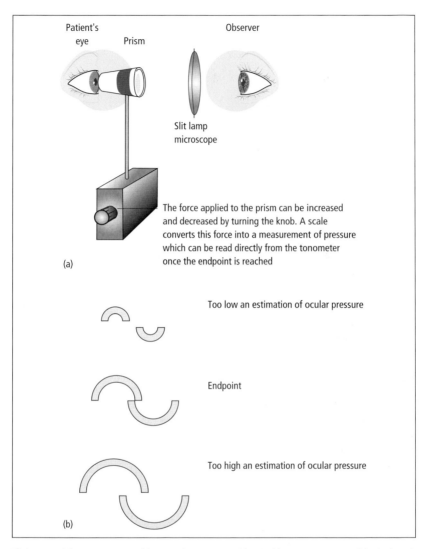

Patient's eye   Prism   Observer

Slit lamp microscope

The force applied to the prism can be increased and decreased by turning the knob. A scale converts this force into a measurement of pressure which can be read directly from the tonometer once the endpoint is reached

(a)

Too low an estimation of ocular pressure

Endpoint

Too high an estimation of ocular pressure

(b)

Figure 2.4 (a) Measurement of intraocular pressure with a Goldmann tonometer. (b) Two hemi-circles are seen by the examiner. The force of contact is increased until the inner borders of the hemicircles just touch. This is the endpoint, at which a fixed amount of flattening of the cornea is achieved.

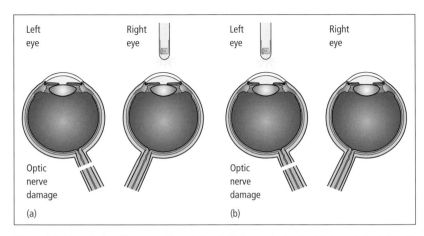

Figure 2.5 The relative afferent pupillary defect (RAPD) or swinging flashlight test. The left optic nerve is damaged. (a) A light shone in the right eye causes both pupils to constrict. (b) When the light is moved to the left eye, both pupils dilate because of the lack of afferent drive to the light reflex; a left relative afferent pupillary defect is present. Opacity of the ocular media (e.g. a dense cataract), or damage to the visual pathway beyond the lateral geniculate body, will not cause a relative afferent pupillary defect.

Where the pupil sizes are equal, in order to test the efferent limb of the pupil reflex, the patient is asked to look at a near object. Normal pupils constrict in conjunction with accommodation and convergence. This is termed *the near reflex*.

The next step is to look for a defect in optic nerve function, using the '*swinging flashlight test*'. This is a sensitive index of an afferent conduction defect. The patient is seated in a dimly illuminated room and views a distant object. A torch is directed at each eye in turn while the pupils are observed. A unilateral defect in optic nerve conduction is demonstrated as a relative afferent pupil defect (RAPD) (see Fig. 2.5 for full description and Chapter 14 for clinical importance). The light is directed at the eye from the side to avoid stimulating the near reflex.

Eye movements

These are assessed while sitting facing the patient. Note the following:
- the position of the eyes;
- the range of eye movements;
- the type of eye movements.

An abnormal direction of one of the eyes in the primary position of gaze (looking straight ahead) may suggest a squint. This can be confirmed by performing a cover test (see Chapter 15).

The range of eye movements is assessed by asking the subject to follow a moving object. Horizontal, vertical and oblique movements are checked from the primary position of gaze, asking the patient to report any double vision (*diplopia*). The presence of oscillating eye movements (*nystagmus*) (see Chapter 15) is also noted. Movement of the eyes when following an object is recorded. Such movements (*pursuit* movements) are usually smooth but may be altered in disease. The ability to direct gaze rapidly from one object to another (*saccadic* eye movements) can be tested by asking the patient to look at targets (such as the finger) held at either side of the head. These movements should be fast, smooth and accurate (that is they should not overshoot or undershoot the target).

Eyelids

These are usually symmetrical in height. The margin of the lid is applied closely to the globe in the healthy eye. If the lid margin is turned away from the globe an *ectropion* is present; if the lid margin is turned in and the lashes are rubbing against the globe an *entropion* is present.

A drooping lid (*ptosis*) may reflect:

- An anatomical disorder (e.g. a congenital or age-related failure of the levator tendon to insert properly into the tarsal plate).
- An organic problem (e.g. weakness of the levator muscle in myasthenia gravis or impairment of its nerve supply in third nerve palsy).

In assessing ptosis, the distance between the upper and lower lids is measured with the patient looking straight ahead. The excursion of the upper lid from extreme downgaze to extreme upgaze is then recorded. In myasthenia, repeated up and down movements of the lids will increase the ptosis by fatiguing the levator muscle (see Chapter 5).

Anatomical examination of the eye

Lids and anterior segment

Simple examination of the eye and adnexae can reveal a great deal about pathological processes within the eye.

Ophthalmologists use a biomicroscope (*slit lamp*) to examine the eye and lids. This allows the examiner to obtain a magnified, stereoscopic view. The slit of light permits a cross-section of the transparent media of the eye to be viewed. By adjusting the angle between this beam and the viewing microscope the light can be used to highlight different structures and pathological processes within the eye. Each structure is carefully examined, starting with the lids and working inwards.

Examination without a slit lamp

Without a slit lamp the eye can still be meaningfully examined with a suitable light. Comment can be made on:
- The conjunctiva: is it injected (inflamed), is there a discharge, what is the distribution of redness, is a conjunctival haemorrhage present?
- The cornea: is it clear, is there a bright reflection of light from the overlying tear film?
- The anterior chamber: is it intact (if penetrating injury is suspected), is a hypopyon present (see Chapter 9)?
- The iris and pupil: is the shape of the pupil normal?
- The lens: is there an opacity in the red reflex observed with the ophthalmoscope?

Diagnostic use of fluorescein

Fluorescein has the property of absorbing light in the blue wavelength and emitting a green fluorescence. The application of fluorescein to the eye can identify corneal abrasions (where the surface epithelial cells have been lost) and leakage of aqueous humour from the eye (Fig. 2.6).

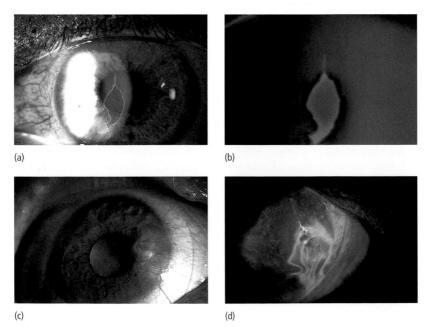

(a)

(b)

(c)

(d)

Figure 2.6 (a) A corneal abrasion (the corneal epithelial layer has been damaged); (b) fluorescein uniformly stains the area of damage. (c) A perforated cornea leaking aqueous (the leak is protected here with a soft contact lens); (d) the fluorescein fluoresces as it is diluted by the leaking aqueous.

To examine an abrasion
- A weak solution of the dye is applied to the eye.
- The eye is examined with a blue light.
- The area of the abrasion will fluoresce bright green.

To determine if fluid is leaking from the eye (e.g. after penetrating corneal injury)
- 2% solution of fluorescein – which is not fluoresent – is applied to the eye.
- The eye is examined with a blue light.
- The dye, diluted by the leaking aqueous, becomes bright green at its junction with the dark, concentrated fluorescein.

Eversion of the upper lid

The underside of the upper lid is examined by everting it over a small blunt-ended object (e.g. a cotton bud) placed in the lid crease (Fig. 2.7). This is an important technique to master as foreign bodies may often lodge under the upper lid, causing considerable pain to the patient.

Retina

The retina is examined by:
- Direct ophthalmoscopy (the conventional ophthalmoscope) (Fig. 2.8).
- Indirect ophthalmoscopy, which allows the extreme retinal periphery to be viewed. The examiner wears a head-mounted binocular microscope with a light source. A lens placed between the examiner and the eye of the subject is used to produce an inverted image of the retina.
- A special contact lens (e.g. a three-mirror lens) is also used at the slit lamp.

The latter two techniques are reserved for specialists; the technique that must be mastered by the non-specialist is direct ophthalmoscopy.

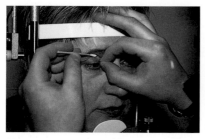 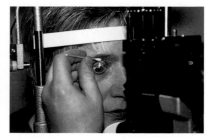

(a)   (b)

Figure 2.7 Eversion of the upper lid using a cotton bud placed in the lid crease.

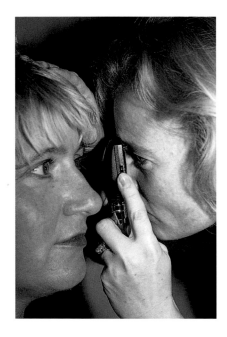

Figure 2.8 The technique of direct ophthalmoscopy. Note that the left eye of the observer is used to examine the left eye of the subject. The closer the observer is to the patient the larger the field of view.

The direct ophthalmoscope provides:
- an image of the red reflex;
- a magnified view of the optic nerve head, macula, retinal blood vessels and the retina to the equator.

It comprises:
- a light source, the size and colour of which can be changed;
- a system of lenses which permits the refractive error of both observer and patient to be corrected.

Confident use of the ophthalmoscope comes with practice. The best results are obtained if the pupil is first dilated with *tropicamide*, a mydriatic with a short duration of action.

The patient and examiner must be comfortable, and the patient looks straight ahead at a distant object. The examiner's right eye is used to examine the patient's right eye, and the left eye to examine the left eye.

The examiner, with the ophthalmoscope about 30 cm away from the eye, views the red reflex through the pupil. The correct power of lens in the ophthalmoscope to produce a clear image is found by ratcheting down from a high to a low hypermetropic (plus) correction. Opacities in the cornea or lens of the eye will appear black against the red reflex. The eye is then approached to within a couple of

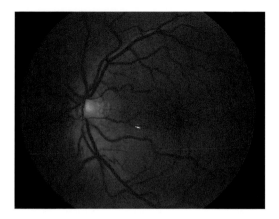

Figure 2.9 A normal left fundus. Note the optic disc with retinal veins and arteries passing from it to branch over the retina. The large temporal vessels form the *temporal arcades*. The macula lies temporal to the disc with the fovea at its centre.

centimetres and the power of the lenses is adjusted in the myopic (minus) direction, to achieve focus on the retina.

The examiner may find it helpful to place a hand on the subject's forehead, which can also be used to hold the upper lid open. The retina should now be in view. It is important to try and examine the retina in a logical sequence so that nothing is overlooked.

● First find the optic disc (Fig. 2.9). Assess its margins (are they indistinct – as in papilloedema?). Assess the colour of the disc (is it pale – as in optic atrophy?). Assess the optic cup (see Chapter 10).

● Examine the macular region. Is there a normal foveal reflex? (In youth the foveal pit appears as a bright pinpoint of light in the centre of the retina.) Are there any abnormal lesions such as haemorrhages, exudates or cotton-wool spots?

● Return to the optic disc and follow each major vessel branch of the vasculature out to the periphery. Are the vessels of normal diameter? Do the arteries nip the veins where they cross (*A/V nipping* – in hypertension)? Are there any emboli in the arterioles? Also examine the surrounding retina for abnormalities.

● Examine the peripheral retina with a 360° sweep.

Direct ophthalmoscopy

● Use an ophthalmoscope with a good illumination.
● Before examining the patient, set the ophthalmoscope power to a low plus, allowing you to focus through from the front to the back of the eye.
● Retinal examination requires that the examiner is close to the subject. An inadequate view will result if the examiner is too far away.
● Where the patient is highly short-sighted, you will find it easier to view the fundi if the patient's spectacles stay in place.
● Practice, practice, practice.

Special examination techniques

Diagnostic lenses

Ophthalmologists employ special lenses that can be used in conjunction with the slit lamp to examine particular ocular structures.

A *gonioscopy* lens is a diagnostic contact lens with a built-in mirror that permits examination of the iridocorneal angle. A larger lens with three mirrors allows the peripheral retina to be seen with the pupil dilated. Both are applied to the anaesthetized cornea with a lubricating medium. Other lenses can be used to obtain a stereoscopic view of the retina.

Retinoscopy

The technique of retinoscopy allows the refractive state of the eye to be measured (i.e. the required strength of a corrective spectacle lens). A streak of light from the retinoscope is directed into the eye. The reflection from the retina is observed through the retinoscope. By gently moving the retinoscope from side to side the reflected image is seen to move. The direction in which this image moves depends on the refractive error of the eye. By placing trial lenses of differing power in front of the eye, the direction in which the reflected image moves is seen to reverse. When this point is reached the refractive error has been determined.

Investigative techniques

Ultrasound

This is used extensively in ophthalmology to provide information about the vitreous, retina and posterior coats of the eye (see Fig. 11.7), particularly when they cannot be clearly visualized (if, for example, there is a dense cataract or vitreous haemorrhage). Ultrasound is also used to measure the length of the eyeball prior to cataract surgery to estimate the power of the artificial lens that is to be implanted into the eye (see Chapter 8).

Keratometry

The shape of the cornea (the radius of curvature) can be measured from the image of a target reflected from its surface. This is important in contact lens assessment (Chapter 3), refractive surgery (Chapter 3) and in calculating the power of an artificial lens implant in cataract surgery (Chapter 8). The technique of photo-keratometry allows a very accurate contour map of the cornea to be produced

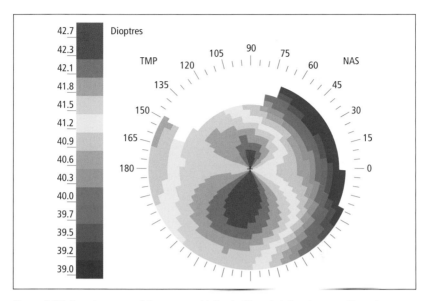

Figure 2.10 A contour map of the cornea obtained with a photokeratoscope. The colours represent areas of different corneal curvature and hence different refractive power.

(Fig. 2.10). These techniques can be used to detect aberrations of shape such as a conical cornea (*keratoconus*).

Synoptophore

This machine permits the assessment of binocular single vision, the ability of the two eyes to work together to produce a single image. It can also assess the range over which the eyes can move away from (*diverge*) or towards each other (*converge*) whilst maintaining a single picture (to measure the range of fusion).

Exophthalmometer

This device measures ocular protrusion (*proptosis*).

Electrophysiological tests

The electrical activity of the retina and visual cortex in response to specific visual stimuli, for example a flashing light, can be used to assess the functioning of the retina (*electroretinogram* or *ERG*), RPE (*electro-oculogram*) and the visual pathway (*visually evoked response* or *potential*).

Radiological imaging techniques

CT and MRI scans have largely replaced skull and orbital X-rays in the imaging of the orbit and visual pathway. The newer diagnostic techniques have enhanced the diagnosis of orbital disease (e.g. optic nerve sheath meningioma) and visual pathway lesions such as pituitary tumours. They have also become the first-line investigation in orbital trauma.

Fluorescein angiography

This technique (Fig. 2.11) provides detailed information about the retinal circulation. Fluorescein dye is injected into the antecubital vein. A *fundus camera* is used to take photographs of the retina. A blue light is directed into the eye to 'excite' the fluorescein in the retinal circulation. The emitted green light is then photographed through a yellow barrier filter which absorbs any reflected blue light.

In this way a fluorescent picture of the retinal circulation is obtained (Fig. 2.12). The dye leaks from abnormal blood vessels (e.g. the new vessels sometimes seen in diabetic eye disease). Areas of ischaemia, due to retinal capillary closure, fail to demonstrate the normal passage of dye (e.g. in a central retinal vein occlusion). The technique is useful both in diagnosis and in planning and following treatment.

Digital imaging and laser scanning techniques

New techniques of retinal imaging are being developed to improve the quality of

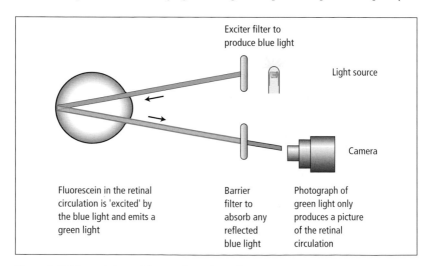

Figure 2.11 The technique of fluorescein angiography.

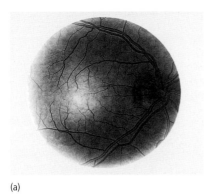
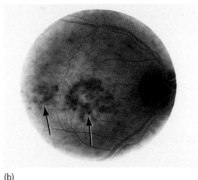

(a)   (b)

Figure 2.12 A fluorescein angiogram. (a) A photograph of the early phase, taken shortly after fluorescein has entered the eye: it can be seen in the choroidal circulation as background fluorescence. (b) In the late phase, some minutes after injection of the dye, areas of hyperfluorescence (the dark areas, arrowed) can be seen around the macula. There has been leakage from abnormal blood vessels into the extravascular tissue space in the macular region (macular oedema).

retinal and optic disc pictures and to permit quantitative assessment of features such as the area of the optic disc and optic disc cup (Chapter 10) and the retina (Chapter 11). These will help in the assessment of patients with chronic diseases such as glaucoma and diabetes, where the management requires an accurate assessment of any change in the disc or retina.

Multiple choice questions

1. Physiological testing of the eye

a The Snellen chart measures visual acuity, the resolving power of the eye.
b The Snellen chart is positioned at 4 metres from the patient.
c The Cardiff Acuity Test relies on preferential looking.
d An isoptre on a visual field chart represents the eye's ability to see a point of light of given size and brightness.
e Intraocular pressure is measured with a perimeter.

2. Pupils

a The term miosis means a constricted pupil.
b Anisocoria means that the pupils differ in size.
c Damage to oculo-motor parasympathetic fibres causes miosis.

d A relative afferent pupillary defect indicates optic nerve disease.
e Normal pupils dilate during convergence.

3. Lids

a When the lid margin is turned away from the eye, this is ectropion.
b When the lid margin is turned into the eye, this is entropion.
c A third nerve palsy may cause ptosis.
d In myasthenia repeated lid blinking increases any ptosis.

4. Fluorescein

a Is excited by green light and emits in the blue wave band.
b Will stain a corneal abrasion.
c To detect its fluorescence, the eye must be examined with a blue light.
d Can be used to demonstrate a leak of aqueous from the anterior chamber.
e Is used to examine the vasculature of the retina.

5. The direct ophthalmoscope

a Produces a magnified image of the retina.
b Contains lenses which increase the magnification.
c Can be used to examine the red reflex.
d The retina can be seen by holding the instrument at a distance of 30 cm from the eye.
e The illumination can be altered.

6. Instruments

a Keratometry allows the protrusion of the eye to be measured.
b The synoptophore measures convergence and divergence.
c The exophthalmometer measure corneal shape.
d Retinoscopy is used to assess refractive error.

Answers

1. Physiological testing of the eye

a True.
b False. The chart is positioned at 6 metres unless mirrors are used.
c True.
d True.

e False. A perimeter measures the visual field. A tonometer measures intraocular pressure.

2. Pupils

a True, mydriasis refers to a dilated pupil.
b True.
c False. Blockade of these parasympathetic fibres results in mydriasis because of the continued sympathetic dilator activity.
d True.
e False. They will constrict.

3. Lids

a True.
b True.
c True.
d True.

4. Fluorescein

a False. Fluorescein is excited by blue light and emits in the green.
b True.
c True.
d True.
e True. This is called fluorescein angiography.

5. The direct ophthalmoscope

a True. The image is magnified some 16 times.
b False. The lenses allow the refractive error of patient and examiner to be corrected.
c True. This is an important part of the examination.
d False. To see the retina the observer must be close to the eye.
e True. The size and colour of the illumination can be altered.

6. Instruments

a False. Keratometry involves the measurement of corneal shape.
b True.
c False. This allows the protrusion of the eye to be measured.
d True.

Chapter 3

Clinical optics

Learning objectives

To understand:
- The different refractive states of the eye, accommodation and presbyopia.
- The means of correcting refractive error in cataract surgery.
- The correction of vision with contact lenses, spectacles and refractive surgery.

Introduction

Light can be defined as that part of the electromagnetic spectrum to which the retina is sensitive. The visible part of the spectrum lies in the waveband of 390 nm to 760 nm. For the eye to generate accurate visual information light must be correctly focused on the retina. The focus must be adjustable to allow equally clear vision of near and distant objects. The cornea, or actually the air/tear interface, is responsible for two-thirds of the focusing power of the eye, and the crystalline lens for one-third. These two refracting elements in the eye converge the rays of light because:

- The cornea has a higher refractive index than air; the lens has a higher refractive index than the aqueous and vitreous humours that surround it. The velocity of light is reduced in a dense medium so that light is refracted towards the normal. When passing from the air to the cornea, or from the aqueous to the lens, the rays therefore converge.
- The refracting surfaces of the cornea and lens are spherically convex.

Ametropia

When parallel rays of light from a distant object are brought to a focus on the retina with the eye at rest (i.e. not accommodating) the refractive state of the eye is known as *emmetropia* (Fig. 3.1). Such an individual can see sharply in the distance without accommodation.

In *ametropia*, parallel rays of light are not brought to a focus on the retina in an eye at rest. A change in refraction is required to achieve sharp vision.

Ametropia may be divided into:

● *Myopia* (short-sightedness): the optical power of the eye is too high (usually due to an elongated globe) and parallel rays of light are brought to a focus in front of the retina (Fig. 3.2).

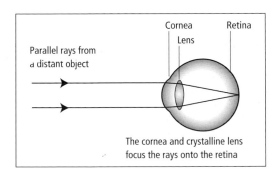

Figure 3.1 The rays of light in an emmetropic eye are focused on the retina.

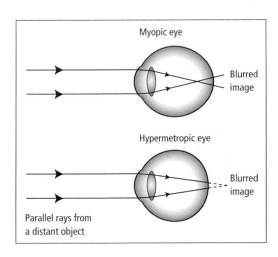

Figure 3.2 Myopia and hypermetropia.

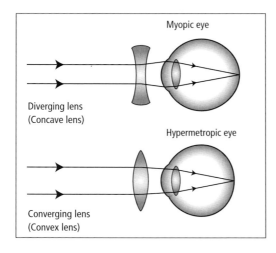

Myopic eye

Diverging lens
(Concave lens)

Hypermetropic eye

Converging lens
(Convex lens)

Figure 3.3 Correction of ametropia with spectacle lenses.

● *Hypermetropia* (long-sightedness): the optical power is too low (usually because the eye is too short) and parallel rays of light converge towards a point behind the retina (Fig. 3.2).

● *Astigmatism*: the optical power of the cornea in different planes is not equal. Parallel rays of light passing through these different planes are brought to different points of focus.

All three types of ametropia can be corrected by spectacle lenses (Fig. 3.3). These diverge the rays in myopia, converge the rays in hypermetropia, and correct for the non-spherical shape of the cornea in astigmatism. It should be noted that in hypermetropia, accommodative effort will bring distant objects into focus by increasing the power of the lens. This will use up the accommodative reserve for near objects.

Accommodation and presbyopia

As an object of regard is brought nearer to the eye, focus is maintained by an increase in the power of the lens of the eye; this is *accommodation* (Fig. 3.4). The eyes also converge.

The ability to accommodate decreases with age, reaching a critical point at about 40-plus years, when the subject experiences difficulty with near vision (*presbyopia*). This occurs earlier in hypermetropes than in myopes. The problem is overcome with convex reading lenses, which provide the converging power no longer supplied by the lens of the eye.

More globular shape
of lens attained with
accommodation

Figure 3.4 The effect of accommodation on the lens.

Optical correction after cataract extraction

The lens provides one-third of the refractive power of the eye, so that after cataract extraction (the removal of an opaque lens) the eye is rendered highly hypermetropic, a condition termed *aphakia*. This can be corrected by:
- the insertion of an intraocular lens at the time of surgery;
- contact lenses;
- aphakic spectacles.

Intraocular lenses give the best optical results. These are placed at the site of the natural lens and mimic its performance. As they are unable to change shape the eye cannot accommodate. An eye with an intraocular lens is said to be *pseudophakic*.

Contact lenses are worn at the surface of the cornea and produce slight magnification of the retinal image (110%); this is not of visual significance. Insertion, removal and cleaning can be difficult for elderly patients or those with physical disability (e.g. arthritis).

Aphakic spectacles have a number of disadvantages:
- They are powerful positive lenses which magnify the retinal image by about 133%, causing the patient to misjudge distances. They cannot be used to correct one eye alone if the other eye is *phakic* (the natural lens is *in situ*) or pseudophakic, because of the disparity in image size between the two corrected eyes (*aniseikonia*). This causes symptoms of dizziness and diplopia.
- Aphakic lenses induce many optical aberrations, including distortion of the image due to the thickness of the lens.

Contact lenses

These are made either from rigid gas-permeable or from soft hydrophilic materials. All contact lenses retard the diffusion of oxygen to the cornea but rigid gas-permeable lenses are relatively more permeable than soft lenses. Although soft lenses are better tolerated physically, gas-permeable lenses have certain advantages:
- Their greater oxygen-permeability reduces the risk of corneal damage from hypoxia.

- Their rigidity allows easier cleaning and offers less risk of infection.
- Their rigidity permits an effective correction of astigmatism.
- Proteinaceous debris is less likely to adhere to the lens and cause an allergic conjunctivitis.

Daily disposable contact lenses are available which are discarded on the day of use.

Soft contact lenses without a refractive function may also be used as ocular *bandages*, e.g. in the treatment of some corneal diseases such as a persistent epithelial defect.

Spectacles

Spectacles are available to correct most refractive errors. Lenses can be made to correct long- and short-sightedness and astigmatism. They are simple and safe to use but may be lost or damaged. Some people find them cosmetically unacceptable and prefer to wear contact lenses. The correction of presbyopia requires additional lens power to overcome the eye's reduced accommodation for near focus. This can be achieved with:

- Separate pairs of glasses for distance and near vision.
- A pair of bifocal lenses, where the near correction is added to the lower segment of the distance lens.
- Varifocal lenses, where the power of the lens gradually changes from the distance correction (in the upper part) to the near correction (in the lower part). This provides sharper middle-distance vision but the lenses may be difficult to manage.

People with particular needs, such as musicians, may also need glasses for middle distance.

Low-vision aids

Patients with poor vision can be helped by advice on lighting conditions and low-vision aids. Clinics specializing in low vision are available in most eye units. Devices used include:

- magnifiers for near vision (Fig. 3.5);
- telescopes for distance vision;
- closed-circuit television to provide magnification and improve contrast;
- large-print books;
- talking clocks and watches;
- a variety of gadgets to help the patient manage household tasks.

Refractive surgery

Although refractive errors are most commonly corrected by spectacles or contact lenses, laser surgical correction is gaining popularity. The excimer laser precisely

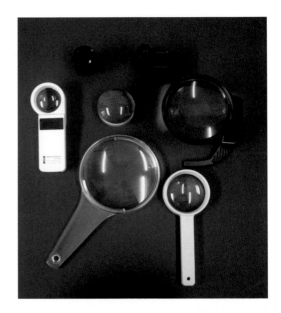

Figure 3.5 Some examples of low-vision aids. Most aid near tasks such as reading. Two monocular telescopes, to help with distance vision, are shown at the top.

removes part of the superficial stromal tissue from the cornea to modify its shape. Myopia is corrected by flattening the cornea and hypermetropia by steepening it. In photorefractive keratectomy (PRK), the laser is applied to the corneal surface having removed the epithelium. In laser-assisted *in situ* keratomileusis (LASIK), a hinged, partial-thickness flap of corneal stroma is first created with a rapidly moving automated blade. The flap is lifted and the laser applied to the stromal bed. The flap is then restored to its original position. Unlike PRK, LASIK provides a near instantaneous improvement in vision with minimal discomfort. Serious complications during flap creation occur rarely. Intraocular lenses can also be placed in a phakic eye to correct severe refractive error, but this carries all the risks of intra-ocular surgery and the possibility of cataract formation.

Multiple choice questions

1. Clinical optics
a The visible spectrum extends from 390 to 760 nm.
b Emmetropia means that parallel rays of light are brought to a focus on the retina when accommodation is relaxed.
c In myopia the rays are focused in front of the retina, in hypermetropia they are focused behind the retina.
d Astigmatism suggests that the cornea is perfectly round.
e Presbyopia refers to the loss of accommodation with age.

2. Correction of ametropia

a A concave lens causes divergence of parallel rays and is used to correct myopia.

b A convex lens causes convergence of parallel rays and is used to correct hypermetropia.

c The natural lens provides 50% of the refractive power of the eye.

d Aphakic spectacles magnify the retinal image.

e The power of the crystalline lens decreases with accommodation.

Answers

1. Clinical optics

a True.

b True.

c True.

d False. It suggests that the shape of the cornea is similar to a rugby ball.

e True.

2. Correction of ametropia

a True.

b True.

c False. It produces about 33% of the refractive power of the eye.

d True. This magnification effect creates optical problems for patients wearing aphakic spectacles.

e False. The power of the lens increases with accommodation.

Chapter 4

The orbit

Learning objectives

To understand the symptoms, signs, investigation and causes of orbital disease.

Introduction

The orbit provides:
- protection to the globe;
- attachments which stabilize the ocular movement;
- transmission of nerves and blood vessels.

Despite the number of different tissues present in the orbit the expression of disease due to different pathologies is often similar.

Clinical features

Proptosis

Proptosis, or *exophthalmos*, is a protrusion of the eye caused by a space-occupying lesion. It can be measured with an exophthalmometer. A difference of more than 3 mm between the two eyes is significant. Various other features give a clue to the pathological process involved (Fig. 4.1).

- If the eye is displaced directly forwards it suggests a lesion that lies within the cone formed by the extraocular muscles (an intra-conal lesion). An example would be an optic nerve sheath meningioma.

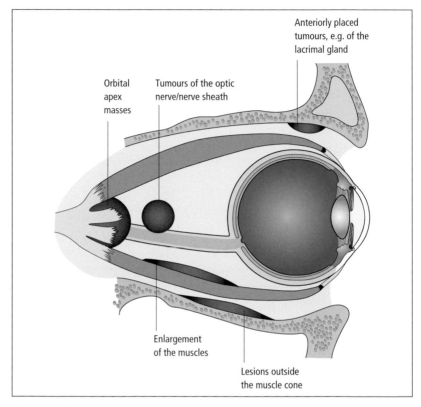

Anteriorly placed
tumours, e.g. of the
lacrimal gland

Orbital
apex
masses

Tumours of the optic
nerve/nerve sheath

Enlargement
of the muscles

Lesions outside
the muscle cone

Figure 4.1 Sites of orbital disease.

- If the eye is displaced to one side a lesion outside the muscle cone is likely (an extra-conal lesion). For example, a tumour of the lacrimal gland displaces the globe to the nasal side.
- A transient proptosis induced by increasing the cephalic venous pressure (by a Valsalva manoeuvre) is a sign of orbital varices.
- The speed of onset of proptosis may also give clues to the aetiology. A slow onset suggests a benign tumour whereas rapid onset is seen in inflammatory disorders, malignant tumours and caroticocavernous sinus fistula.
- The presence of pain may suggest infection (e.g. orbital cellulitis).

Enophthalmos

Enophthalmos is a backward displacement of the globe. This may be seen following an orbital fracture when orbital contents are displaced into an adjacent sinus. It is also said to occur in Horner's syndrome, but this is really a pseudo-enophthalmos due to narrowing of the palpebral fissure (see Chapter 13).

Pain

Inflammatory conditions, infective disorders and rapidly progressing tumours cause pain. This is not usually present with benign tumours.

Eyelid and conjunctival changes

Conjunctival injection and swelling suggest an inflammatory or infective process. Infection is associated with reduced eye movements, erythema and swelling of the lids (*orbital cellulitis*). With more anterior lid inflammation (*preseptal cellulitis*), eye movements are full.

Florid engorgement of the conjunctival vessels suggests a vascular lesion caused by the development of a fistula between the carotid artery and the cavernous sinus.

Diplopia

Diplopia occurs when only one eye is directed at the object of regard, due to:
- Direct involvement of the muscles in *myositis* and *dysthyroid eye disease* (Graves' Disease). Movement is restricted in a direction opposite to the field of action of the affected muscle. The eye appears to be tethered (e.g. if the inferior rectus is thickened in thyroid eye disease there will be restriction of upgaze).
- Involvement of the nerve supply to the extraocular muscles. Here diplopia occurs during gaze into the field of action of the muscle (e.g. palsy of the right lateral rectus produces diplopia in right horizontal gaze).

Visual acuity

This may be reduced by:
- exposure keratopathy from severe proptosis, when the cornea is no longer protected by the lids and tear film;
- optic nerve involvement by compression or inflammation;
- distortion of the macula due to posterior compression of the globe by a space-occupying lesion.

Investigation of orbital disease

CT and MRI scans have greatly helped in the diagnosis of orbital disease – localizing the site of the lesion, demonstrating enlarged intraocular muscles in dysthyroid eye disease and myositis, or visualizing fractures to the orbit. Additional systemic tests will be dictated by the differential diagnosis (e.g. tests to determine the primary site of a secondary tumour).

Differential diagnosis of orbital disease

(Traumatic orbital disease is discussed in Chapter 16.)

Disorders of the extraocular muscles

Dysthyroid eye disease and *ocular myositis* present with symptoms and signs of orbital disease. They are described in Chapter 15.

In children a rapidly developing proptosis may be caused by a rare *rhabdomyosarcoma* arising from the extraocular muscles (see Orbital tumours, below).

Infective disorders

Orbital cellulitis is a serious condition which can cause blindness and may spread to cause a brain abscess (Fig. 4.2). The infection often arises from an adjacent ethmoid sinus. The commonest causative organism is *Haemophilus influenzae*. The patient presents with:

- a painful eye;
- periorbital inflammation and swelling;
- reduced eye movements;
- conjunctival injection;
- possible visual loss;
- systemic illness and pyrexia.

An MRI or CT scan is helpful in diagnosis and in planning treatment. The condition usually responds to intravenous broad-spectrum antibiotics, but it may be necessary to drain an abscess or decompress the orbit, particularly if the optic

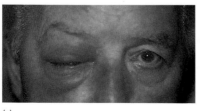

(a)

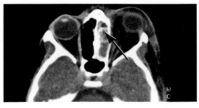

(b)

Figure 4.2 (a) The clinical appearance of a patient with right orbital cellulitis. (b) A CT scan showing a left opaque ethmoid sinus and subperiosteal orbital abscess.

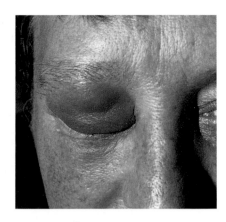

Figure 4.3 The appearance of a patient with preseptal cellulitis.

nerve is compromised. Optic nerve function must be watched closely, checking acuity, monitoring colour vision and testing for a relative afferent pupillary defect. Orbital decompression is usually performed with the help of an ENT specialist.

A preseptal cellulitis involves only the lid (Fig. 4.3). It presents with periorbital inflammation and swelling but not the other ocular features of orbital cellulitis. Eye movement is not impaired.

An orbital mucocoele arises from accumulated secretions within any of the paranasal sinuses when natural drainage of the sinus is blocked. Surgical excision may be required.

Inflammatory disease

The orbit may become involved in various inflammatory disorders, including sarcoidosis and orbital pseudotumour, a non-specific lymphofibroblastic disorder. Diagnosis of such conditions is difficult. The presence of other systemic signs of sarcoidosis may be helpful. If an orbital pseudotumour is suspected it may be necessary to biopsy the tissue to differentiate the lesion from a lymphoma.

Vascular abnormalities

A fistula may develop in the cavernous sinus between the carotid artery or a dural artery and the cavernous sinus itself (*caroticocavernous sinus fistula*). This causes the veins to be exposed to an intravascular high pressure. The eye is proptosed and the conjunctival veins dilated. The patient may complain of a pulsatile tinnitus. A bruit may be heard with a stethoscope over the eye in time with the radial pulse. Extraocular muscle engorgement reduces eye movements, and increased pressure in the veins draining the eye causes an increased intraocular pressure. Interventional

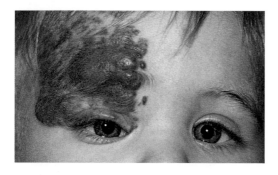

Figure 4.4 The appearance of a capillary haemangioma.

radiological techniques can be used to close the fistula by embolizing and throm-bosing the affected vascular segment.

The orbital veins may become dilated (*orbital varix*), causing intermittent prop-tosis when venous pressure is raised.

In infants, a *capillary haemangioma* may present as an extensive lesion of the orbit and the surrounding skin (Fig. 4.4). Fortunately most undergo spontaneous resolution in the first five years of life. Treatment is indicated if size or position obstructs the visual axis and risks the development of amblyopia (see Chapter 15). Local injection of steroids is usually successful in reducing the size of the lesion.

Orbital tumours

The following tumours may produce signs of orbital disease:
- lacrimal gland tumours;
- optic nerve gliomas;
- meningiomas;
- lymphomas;
- rhabdomyosarcoma;
- metastasis from other systemic cancers (neuroblastomas in children, the breast, lung, prostate or gastrointestinal tract in adults).

A CT or MRI scan will help with the diagnosis (Fig. 4.5). Again systemic investiga-tion, for example to determine the site of a primary tumour, may be required.

Malignant *lacrimal gland tumours* carry a poor prognosis. Benign tumours still require complete excision to prevent malignant transformation. Optic nerve *gliomas* may be associated with *neurofibromatosis*. They are difficult to treat but are often slow-growing and thus may require no intervention. *Meningiomas* of the optic nerve are rare, and may also be difficult to excise. Again they can be observed, and some may benefit from treatment with radiotherapy. Meningiomas from the middle cranial fossa may spread through the optic canal into the orbit. The

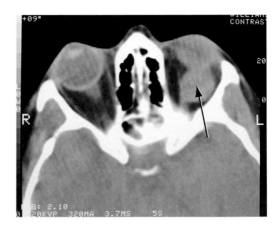

Figure 4.5 A CT scan showing a left-sided orbital secondary tumour.

treatment of *lymphoma* requires a full systemic investigation to determine whether the lesion is indicative of widespread disease or whether it is localized to the orbit. In the former case the patient is treated with chemotherapy, in the latter with localized radiotherapy.

In children the commonest orbital tumour is a *rhabdomyosarcoma*, a rapidly growing tumour of striated muscle. Chemotherapy is effective if the disease is localized to the orbit.

Dermoid cysts

These congenital lesions are caused by the continued growth of ectodermal tissue beneath the surface, which may present in the medial or lateral aspect of the superior orbit (Fig. 4.6). Excision is usually performed for cosmetic reasons and to avoid traumatic rupture, which may cause scarring. Some may be attached deeply by a stalk, and a CT scan may be necessary before surgery to identify this deeper connection. Dermoids may also occur at the limbus.

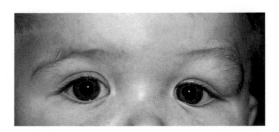

Figure 4.6 A left dermoid cyst.

> ## Key points
> • Suspect orbital cellulitis in a patient with periorbital and conjunctival inflammation, particularly when there is severe pain and the patient is systemically unwell.
> • The commonest cause of bilateral proptosis is dysthyroid disease.
> • The commonest cause of unilateral proptosis is also dysthyroid disease.
> • Dysthyroid disease may be associated with the serious complications of exposure keratopathy and optic nerve compression.

Multiple choice questions

1. A 56-year-old female patient presents with a proptosed eye, deviated nasally.

a An eye displaced to one side of the orbit suggests an extra-conal lesion.

b Rapid onset of proptosis might suggest a malignant tumour.

c The patient may have dysthyroid eye (Graves') disease.

d The patient may have a rhabdomyosarcoma of the extraocular muscles.

e Diplopia is a common presenting feature of orbital disease.

2. A 16-year-old boy presents with swollen eyelids, a red eye, proptosis, severe eye pain and tenderness and a pyrexia. The vision has become very blurred and colour vision is reduced.

a Orbital cellulitis is the most likely diagnosis.

b A relative afferent pupillary defect may be present.

c No investigations are necessary.

d Urgent orbital decompression is indicated.

3. A 70-year-old woman with a history of previous head trauma presents with sudden onset of a red, proptosed eye. Eye movements are reduced in all directions. Vision is intact. Intraocular pressure is increased. The most likely diagnosis is:

a Dysthyroid eye (Graves') disease.

b A caroticocavernous sinus fistula.

c An orbital varix.

d A dermoid cyst.

Answers

1. A 56-year-old female patient presents with a proptosed eye, deviated nasally.

a True.

b True.
c True.
d False. This is seen in much younger patients.
e True.

2. A 16-year-old boy presents with swollen eyelids, a red eye, proptosis, severe eye pain and tenderness and a pyrexia. The vision has become very blurred and colour vision is reduced.
a True. These are the classic symptoms.
b True. The reduced acuity and colour vision suggests that the optic nerve is compromised, so that a relative afferent pupillary defect is expected.
c False. An urgent CT of the orbit should be undertaken to confirm the diagnosis. Blood cultures may also be helpful.
d True. Successful decompression may save optic nerve function.

3. A 70-year-old woman with a history of previous head trauma presents with sudden onset of a red, proptosed eye. Eye movements are reduced in all directions. Vision is intact. Intraocular pressure is increased.
a False. While possible, it is not the most likely diagnosis.
b True. These are the classic features, including the history of trauma.
c False. A varix causes an intermittent proptosis, worsened by an elevated venous pressure, such as may occur with a Valsalva manoeuvre.
d False. Dermoid cysts occur in a much younger age group. They do not cause proptosis and usually present as a swelling at the medial or lateral aspect of the orbit.

Chapter 5

The eyelids

Learning objectives

To understand:
- The symptoms, signs and causes of abnormal eyelid position.
- The symptoms, signs and treatment of blepharitis.
- The causes of lid swellings.

Introduction

The eyelids are important both in providing physical protection to the eyes and in ensuring a normal tear film and tear drainage. Diseases of the eyelids can be divided into those associated with:
- abnormal lid position;
- inflammation of the lid;
- lid lumps;
- abnormalities of the lashes.

Abnormalities of lid position

Ptosis

This is an abnormally low position of the upper eyelid (Fig. 5.1).

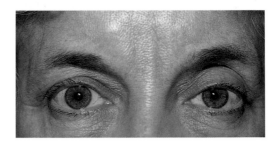

Figure 5.1 Left ptosis.

Pathogenesis

It may be caused by:
1 Mechanical factors.
   a Large lid lesions pulling down the lid.
   b Lid oedema.
   c Tethering of the lid by conjunctival scarring.
   d Structural abnormalities, including a disinsertion of the aponeurosis of the levator muscle, usually in elderly patients.
2 Neurological factors.
   a Third nerve palsy (see Chapter 15).
   b Horner's syndrome, due to a sympathetic nerve lesion (see Chapter 13).
   c Marcus–Gunn jaw-winking syndrome. In this congenital ptosis there is a miswiring of the nerve supply to the pterygoid muscle of the jaw and the levator of the eyelid so that the eyelid moves in conjunction with movements of the jaw.
3 Myogenic factors.
   a Myasthenia gravis (see Chapter 15).
   b Some forms of muscular dystrophy.
   c Chronic external ophthalmoplegia.

Symptoms

Patients present because:
- they object to the cosmetic effect;
- vision may be impaired;
- there are symptoms and signs associated with the underlying cause (e.g. asymmetric pupils in Horner's syndrome, diplopia and reduced eye movements in a third nerve palsy).

Signs

There is a reduction in size of the interpalpebral aperture. The upper lid margin, which usually overlaps the upper limbus by 1–2 mm, may be partially covering the pupil. The function of the levator muscle can be tested by measuring the maximum travel of the upper lid from full upgaze to full downgaze (normally 15–18 mm). Pressure on the brow (frontalis muscle) during this test will prevent its contribution to lid elevation. If myasthenia is suspected the ptosis should be observed during repeated lid movement. Increasing ptosis after repeated elevation and depression of the lid is suggestive of myasthenia. Other underlying signs, for example of Horner's syndrome or a third nerve palsy, may be present.

Management

It is important to exclude an underlying cause whose treatment could resolve the problem (e.g. myasthenia gravis). Ptosis otherwise requires surgical correction. In very young children this is usually deferred, but may be expedited if pupil cover threatens to induce amblyopia.

Entropion

This is an inturning, usually of the lower lid, towards the globe (Fig. 5.2). It may occur if the patient looks downwards or be induced by forced lid closure. It is seen most commonly in elderly patients where the orbicularis muscle becomes weakened. It may also be caused by conjunctival scarring distorting the lid (*cicatricial entropion*). The inturned lashes cause irritation of the eye and may also abrade the cornea. The eye may be red. Short-term treatment includes the application of lubricants to the eye or taping of the lid to overcome the inturning. Permanent treatment requires surgery.

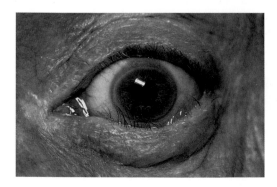

Figure 5.2 Entropion.

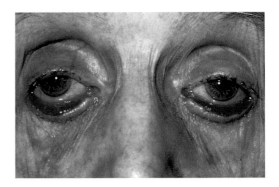

Figure 5.3 Ectropion.

Ectropion

Here there is an eversion of the lid away from the globe (Fig. 5.3). Usual causes include:

- age-related orbicularis muscle laxity;
- scarring of the periorbital skin;
- seventh nerve palsy.

The malposition of the lids everts the puncta and prevents drainage of the tears, leading to epiphora. It also exposes the conjunctiva (see Chapter 6). This also results in an irritable eye. Treatment is again surgical.

Inflammations of the eyelids

Blepharitis

This is a very common, chronic inflammation of the lid margins (Fig. 5.4). In *anterior blepharitis* inflammation of the lid margin is concentrated in the lash line and accompanied by squamous debris around the eyelashes. The conjunctiva becomes injected. It is sometimes associated with a chronic staphylococcal infection. In severe disease the cornea is affected (*blepharokeratitis*). Small infiltrates ulcers may form in the peripheral cornea (*marginal teratitis*) due to an immune complex response to staphylococcal exotoxins.

In *posterior blepharitis* (or *meibomian gland dysfunction*) the meibomian glands are usually obstructed. The two forms may occur independently.

Symptoms

These include:

- tired, itchy, sore eyes, worse in the morning;
- crusting of the lid margins.

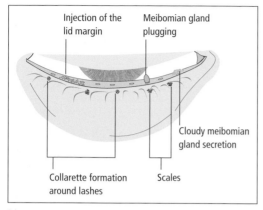

(a)

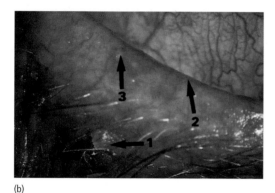

(b)

Figure 5.4 Blepharitis: (a) a diagram showing the signs; (b) the clinical appearance of the lid margin. Note (1) the scales on the lashes, (2) dilated blood vessels on the lid margin and (3) plugging of the meibomian glands.

Signs

In anterior blepharitis there may be:
- redness and scaling of the lid margins;
- debris in the form of a collarette around the eyelashes: some lash bases may be ulcerated – a sign of staphylococcal infection;
- a reduction in the number of eyelashes.

In posterior blepharitis there may be:
- obstruction and plugging of the meibomian orifices;
- thickened, cloudy, expressed meibomian secretions;
- injection of the lid margin and conjunctiva;
- tear film abnormalities and punctate keratitis.

Both forms of blepharitis are strongly associated with seborrhoeic dermatitis, atopic eczema and acne rosacea. In rosacea there is hyperaemia and telangiectasia of the facial skin and a rhinophima (a bulbous irregular swelling of the nose with hypertrophy of the sebaceous glands).

Treatment

This is often difficult and must be long-term.

For anterior blepharitis, lid toilet with a cotton bud wetted with bicarbonate solution or diluted baby shampoo helps to remove squamous debris from the lash line. Topical steroids can reduce inflammation but must be used infrequently, to avoid steroid complications. Staphylococcal lid disease may also require therapy with topical antibiotics (e.g. fusidic acid gel), and occasionally with systemic antibiotics.

For meibomian gland dysfunction, abnormal secretions can be expressed by lid massage after hot bathing through the closed lids. If this treatment fails, then meibomian gland function can be improved by short courses of oral tetracycline. Where meibomian gland obstruction is extensive, the absence of an oily layer on the tear film can induce an evaporative dry eye, which requires treatment with artificial tears.

Prognosis

Although symptoms may be ameliorated by treatment, blepharitis may remain a chronic problem.

Benign lid lumps and bumps

Chalazion

This is a common painless condition in which an obstructed meibomian gland causes a granuloma within the tarsal plate (Fig. 5.5). Symptoms are of an unsightly lid swelling which usually resolves within six months. If the lesion persists it can be incised and the gelatinous contents curetted from the conjunctival surface.

An abscess (*internal hordeolum*) may also form within the meibomian gland. Unlike a chalazion, this is painful. It may respond to topical antibiotics but incision may be necessary.

A stye (*external hordeolum*) is an exquisitely painful abscess of an eyelash follicle. Treatment requires the removal of the associated eyelash and application of hot compresses. Most cases are self-limiting, but occasionally systemic antibiotics are required.

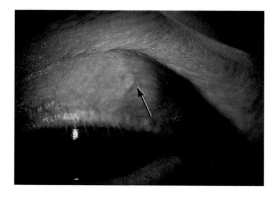

Figure 5.5 Chalazion.

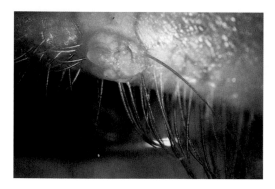

Figure 5.6 Molluscum contagiosum.

Molluscum contagiosum

This umbilicated lesion found on the lid margin is caused by a pox virus (Fig. 5.6). It causes irritation of the eye. The eye is red, and small elevations of lymphoid tissue are found on the tarsal conjunctiva (*follicular conjunctivitis*). Treatment requires excision of the lid lesion.

Cysts

Various cysts may form on the eyelids. Sebaceous cysts are opaque. They rarely cause symptoms. They can be excised for cosmetic reasons. A cyst of Moll is a small translucent cyst on the lid margin caused by obstruction of a sweat gland. A cyst of Zeis is an opaque cyst on the eyelid margin caused by blockage of an accessory sebaceous gland. These can be excised for cosmetic reasons.

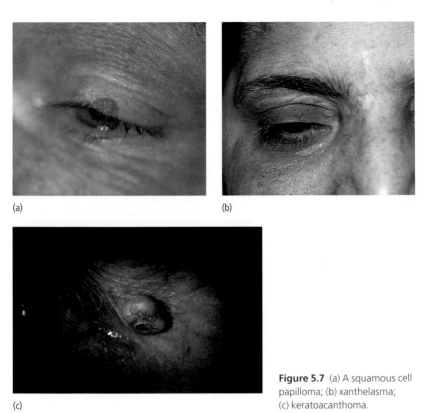

(a)

(b)

(c)

Figure 5.7 (a) A squamous cell papilloma; (b) xanthelasma; (c) keratoacanthoma.

Squamous cell papilloma

This is a common frond-like lid lesion with a fibrovascular core and thickened squamous epithelium (Fig. 5.7a). It is usually asymptomatic but can be excised for cosmetic reasons with cautery to the base.

Xanthelasmas

These are lipid-containing bilateral lesions which may in youth be associated with hypercholesterolaemia (Fig. 5.7b). It is worth checking the blood cholesterol. They are excised for cosmetic reasons.

Keratoacanthoma

A brownish pink, fast-growing lesion with a central crater filled with keratin

(Fig. 5.7c). Treatment is by excision. Careful histology must be performed as some may have the malignant features of a squamous cell carcinoma (see below).

Naevus (mole)

These lesions are derived from naevus cells (altered melanocytes) and can be pigmented or non-pigmented. No treatment is necessary.

Malignant tumours

Basal cell carcinoma

This is the most common form of malignant tumour (Fig. 5.8). Ten per cent of cases occur in the eyelids and account for 90% of eyelid malignancies. The tumour is:

- slow-growing;
- locally invasive;
- non-metastasizing.

Patients present with a painless lesion on the eyelid which may be nodular, sclerosing or ulcerative (the so-called *rodent ulcer*). Typically, it has a pale, pearly margin. A high index of suspicion is required. Treatment is by:

- Excision biopsy with a margin of normal tissue surrounding the lesion. Excision may also be controlled with frozen sections when serial histological assessment is used to determine the need for additional tissue removal (Mohs surgery). This minimizes destruction of normal tissue.
- Cryotherapy.
- Radiotherapy.

The prognosis is usually very good, but deep invasion of the tumour can be difficult to treat.

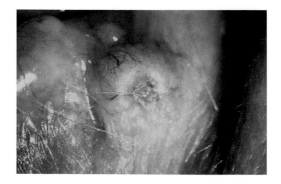

Figure 5.8 A basal cell carcinoma.

Squamous cell carcinoma

This is a less common but more malignant tumour which can metastasize to the lymph nodes. It can arise *de novo* or from pre-malignant lesions. It may present as a hard nodule or a scaly patch. Treatment is by excisional biopsy with a margin of healthy tissue.

UV exposure is an important risk factor for both basal cell and squamous cell carcinoma.

Abnormalities of the lashes

Trichiasis

This is a common condition in which aberrant eyelashes are directed backwards towards the globe. It is distinct from entropion. The lashes rub against the cornea and cause irritation and abrasion. It may result from any cicatricial process. In developing countries trachoma (see Chapter 7) is an important cause and trichiasis is an important basis for the associated blindness. Treatment is by epilation of the offending lashes. Recurrence can be treated with cryotherapy or electrolysis. Any underlying abnormality of lid position needs surgical correction.

Key points

- Blepharitis is a common cause of sore 'tired' irritable eyes.
- A patient with a lid lump and a sore red eye may have molluscum contagiosum.
- Abnormalities of eyelid position can cause corneal disease.
- Always consider the possibility of malignancy in lid lesions.

Multiple choice questions

1. A 55-year-old woman presents with a small ptosis, and miosis on the same side. She is a smoker. The likely diagnosis is

a Myasthenia gravis.

b Marcus–Gunn syndrome.

c Horner's syndrome.

d Third nerve palsy.

e Conjunctival scarring.

2. Blepharitis is associated with

a Cloudy meibomian secretions in posterior blepharitis.

b Injection of the lid margin.

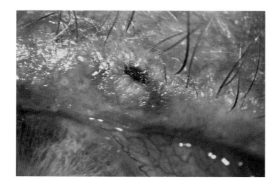

Figure 5.9 The clinical appearance of the eye referred to in Question 3.

c Marginal keratitis.
d An inturned eyelid.
e Debris around the base of an eyelash is termed a rosette.

3. A 70-year-old patient presents with the single lesion shown in Fig. 5.9. It is slowly increasing in size. The most likely diagnosis is
a Keratoacanthoma.
b Basal cell carcinoma.
c Squamous cell carcinoma.
d Molluscum contagiosum.
e Xanthelasma.

Answers

1. A 55-year-old woman presents with a small ptosis, and miosis on the same side. She is a smoker.
a False.
b False.
c True. There is an interruption of the sympathetic supply to the iris dilator and to the smooth muscle of the upper lid. In this patient this may be caused by a tumour of the lung.
d False.
e False.

2. Blepharitis is associated with
a True.
b True.
c True. In anterior blepharitis; due to staphylococcal sensitization.

d False. There is no association between blepharitis and entropion.

e True. This is a feature of anterior blepharitis.

3. A 70-year-old patient presents with the single lesion shown in Fig. 5.9. It is slowly increasing in size.

a False. There is no central crater filled with keratin.

b True. Slow growth is usual, the shape is typical and the pearly margin is also characteristic.

c False. The appearance differs and the condition is less common. It can however metastasize and must be considered in the differential diagnosis.

d False. These lesions are usually umbilicated and may be associated with a red eye and tarsal follicles.

e False. These lipid-laden lesions are usually bilateral and they are not ulcerated.

Chapter 6

The lacrimal system

Learning objectives

To understand:
- The symptoms, signs, causes and treatment of dry eyes.
- The symptoms, signs, causes and treatment of watery eyes.

Introduction

Disorders of the lacrimal system are common and may produce chronic symptoms with a significant morbidity. The lacrimal glands normally produce about 1.2 µl of tears per minute. Some tears are lost by evaporation, while the remainder are drained via the nasolacrimal system. The tear film is re-formed with each blink.

Abnormalities are found in:
- tear flow and evaporation;
- the drainage of tears.

Abnormalities in tear flow and evaporation – dry eye

Dry eye is a condition of the ocular surface due to a deficiency of tear quantity or composition or excessive evaporation, characterized by hyperosmolarity and leading to ocular surface damage, inflammation and symptoms of discomfort and visual loss. An alternative term is *keratoconjunctivitis sicca* (*KCS*).

Aqueous-deficient dry eye

A deficiency of lacrimal secretion occurs with age and may be sufficient to cause dry eyes. When dry eyes occur in combination with a dry mouth and dryness of other mucous membranes the condition is called primary *Sjögren's syndrome* (an autoimmune *exocrinopathy*). When Sjögren's syndrome occurs in association with a specific autoimmune connective-tissue disorder the condition is called secondary Sjögren's syndrome. Rheumatoid arthritis is the commonest of these associated disorders.

Symptoms

Patients have non-specific symptoms of grittiness, burning, photophobia, heaviness of the lids and ocular fatigue. Symptoms are worse in the evening because the eyes dry progressively during the day. In more severe cases visual acuity may be reduced by corneal damage.

Signs

In mild cases there are few obvious signs. Staining of the eye with fluorescein will show small dots of fluorescence (*punctate staining*) over the exposed corneal and conjunctival surfaces. In severe cases (Fig. 6.1) tags of abnormal mucus may attach to the corneal surface (*filamentary keratitis*), causing pain due to tugging on these filaments during blinking.

Treatment

Supplementation of the tears with tear substitutes helps to reduce symptoms, and a humid environment can be created around the eyes with shielded spectacles. In severe cases it may be necessary to occlude the puncta with plugs, or more permanently with surgery, to conserve the tears. Topical anti-inflammatory agents are also in use.

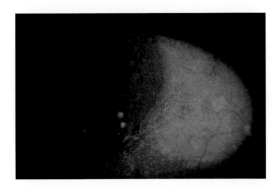

Figure 6.1 Fluorescein staining of cornea and conjunctiva in a severe dry eye.

Prognosis

Mild disease usually responds to artificial tears and tear conservation. Severe disease such as that in rheumatoid Sjögren's can be very difficult to treat.

Evaporative dry eye – inadequate meibomian oil delivery

Extensive meibomian gland obstruction may result in a deficient tear film lipid layer and lead to increased water loss from the eyes. This may exacerbate an existing aqueous-deficient dry eye. Treatment of the meibomian gland dysfunction (posterior blepharitis) is covered in Chapter 5.

Evaporative dry eye – malposition of the globe or lid margins

If the lids are not adequately apposed to the eye (*ectropion*), or there is incomplete lid closure (*lagophthalmos* – e.g. in a seventh nerve palsy), or if the eye protrudes (*proptosis*) as in dysthyroid eye disease, then the preocular tear film will not form adequately and an evaporative form of dry eye will result.

Correction of the lid deformity is required for ectropion. In other instances, if the defect is temporary, artificial tears and lubricants can be applied. If lid closure is inadequate a temporary ptosis can be induced with a local injection of botulinum toxin into the levator muscle. A more permanent result can be obtained by suturing together part of the apposed margins of the upper and lower lids (e.g. *lateral tarsorrhaphy*; Fig. 6.2).

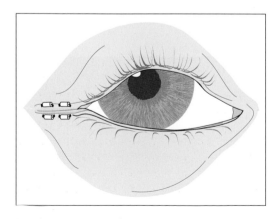

Figure 6.2 A lateral tarsorrhaphy protects a previously exposed cornea.

Inadequate mucus production

Loss of goblet cells occurs in most forms of dry eye, but particularly in cicatricial conjunctival disorders such as erythema multiforme (Stevens–Johnson syndrome). In this there is an acute episode of inflammation causing macular 'target' lesions on the skin and discharging lesions on the eye, mouth and vulva. In the eye this causes conjunctival shrinkage with adhesions forming between the globe and the conjunctiva (*symblepharon*). There may be both an aqueous and a mucin deficiency, and problems due to lid deformity and trichiasis. Chemical burns of the eye, particularly by alkalis, and trachoma (chronic inflammation of the conjunctiva caused by chlamydial infection; see Chapters 7 and 17) may have a similar end result.

The symptoms are similar to those seen with an aqueous deficiency. Examination may reveal scarred, abnormal conjunctiva and areas of fluorescein staining on the cornea. Treatment requires the application of artificial lubricants.

Vitamin A deficiency (*xerophthalmia*) is a condition causing childhood blindness on a worldwide scale. It is associated with generalized malnutrition in countries such as India and Pakistan. Goblet cells are lost from the conjunctiva and the ocular surface becomes keratinized (*xerosis*). An aqueous deficiency may also occur. The characteristic corneal melting and perforation which occur in this condition (*keratomalacia*) may be prevented by early treatment with vitamin A (see Chapter 17 for a more detailed description).

Disorders of tear drainage

When tear production exceeds the capacity of the drainage system, excess tears overflow onto the cheeks. It may be caused by:
- irritation of the ocular surface, e.g. by a corneal foreign body, infection or blepharitis;
- occlusion of any part of the drainage system (when the tearing is termed *epiphora*).

Obstruction of tear drainage (infantile)

The nasolacrimal system develops as a solid cord which subsequently canalizes and is patent just before term. Congenital obstruction of the duct is common. The distal end of the nasolacrimal duct may remain imperforate, causing a watering eye. If the canaliculi also become partially obstructed, the non-draining pool of fluid in the sac may become infected and accumulate within a *mucocoele* or cause *dacrocystitis*. Diagnostically, the discharge may be expressed from the puncta by pressure over the lacrimal sac. The conjunctiva, however, is not inflamed. Most obstructions resolve spontaneously in the first year of life. If epiphora persists beyond this time, patency can be achieved by passing a probe via the punctum through the nasolacrimal duct to perforate the occluding membrane (*probing*). A general anaesthetic is required.

Obstruction of tear drainage (adult)

The tear drainage system may become blocked at any point, although the most common site is the nasolacrimal duct. Causes include infections or direct trauma to the nasolacrimal system.

History

The patient complains of a watering eye, sometimes associated with stickiness. The eye is white. Symptoms may be worse in the wind or in cold weather. There may be a history of previous trauma or infection.

Signs

A stenosed punctum may be apparent on slit lamp examination. Epiphora is unusual if one punctum continues to function. Acquired obstruction beyond the punctum is diagnosed by syringing the nasolacrimal system with saline, using a fine cannula inserted into a canaliculus. A patent system is indicated when the patient tastes the saline as it reaches the pharynx. If there is an obstruction of the nasolacrimal duct then fluid will regurgitate from the non-cannulated punctum. The exact location of the obstruction can be confirmed by injecting a radio-opaque dye into the nasolacrimal system (*dacrocystogram*). X-rays are then used to follow the passage of the dye through the system.

Treatment

It is important to exclude other ocular disease that may contribute to watering, such as blepharitis. Repair of the occluded nasolacrimal duct requires surgery to connect the mucosal surface of the lacrimal sac to the nasal mucosa by removing the intervening bone (*dacryocystorhinostomy* or *DCR*; Fig. 6.3). The operation can be performed through an incision on the side of the nose but it may also be performed endoscopically through the nasal passages, thus avoiding a scar on the face.

Infections of the nasolacrimal system

Closed obstruction of the drainage system predisposes to infection of the sac (*dacryocystitis*; Fig. 6.4). The organism involved is usually *Staphylococcus*. Patients

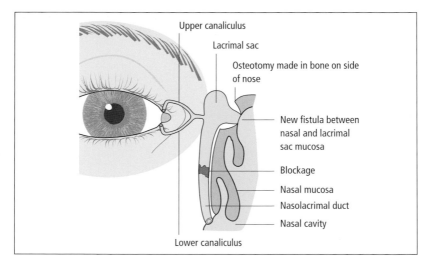

Figure 6.3 The principle of a DCR (dacryocystorhinostomy).

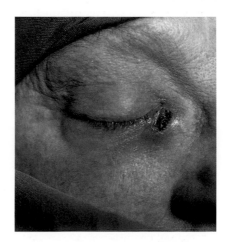

Figure 6.4 Dacryocystitis, unusually, in this case, pointing through the skin.

present with a painful swelling on the medial side of the orbit, which is the enlarged, infected sac. Treatment is with systemic antibiotics. A *mucocoele* results from a collection of mucus in an obstructed sac; it is not grossly infected and is often painless. In either case a DCR may be necessary to prevent recurrence.

> **Key points**
>
> ● Dry eyes can cause significant ocular symptoms and signs.
> ● A watery eye in a newborn child is commonly due to non-patency of the nasolacrimal duct. Most spontaneously resolve within the first year of life.
> ● In an adult a watery eye is due either to excessive lacrimation or dysfunction or blockage of the tear drainage system.

Multiple choice questions

1. Sjögren's syndrome is associated with
a Keratoconjunctivitis sicca (KCS – dry eye).
b Rheumatoid arthritis.
c Cardiac failure.
d Dryness of the mouth.
e Staining of the cornea with fluorescein.

2. A 60-year-old man presents with painless watering of the eye, worse when outside in the wind. Sometimes there is a sticky discharge. The white of the eye is never inflamed. No abnormal masses are palpable, but pressure over the lacrimal sac causes a mucopurulent discharge to be expressed from the lower punctum.
a The most likely diagnosis is an ectropion.
b The most likely diagnosis is a blocked nasolacrimal duct.
c The site of a nasolacrimal obstruction can be confirmed with a dacrocystogram.
d The most likely diagnosis is blepharitis.
e The most likely diagnosis is dacrocystitis.

Answers

1. Sjögren's syndrome
a True.
b True. The association with connective tissue disease is called secondary Sjögren's syndrome.
c False.
d True. Dry eye and dry mouth are key features of Sjögren's syndrome.
e True. Dry eye damages the corneal (and conjunctival) epithelium.

2. A 60-year-old man presents with painless watering of the eye, worse when outside in the wind.
a False. This may cause epiphora, but there would not usually be a discharge,

nor would there be a mucopurulent discharge expressed from the lower punctum.

b True. The symptoms and signs are typical of the condition.

c True. The radio-opaque dye outlines the nasolacrimal system.

d False. Although blepharitis can cause epiphora there would be no mucopurulent discharge expressible from the lower punctum.

e False. There is no swelling over the lacrimal sac.

Chapter 7

Conjunctiva, cornea and sclera

Learning objectives

To understand:
- The symptoms, signs, causes and treatment of conjunctival disease.
- The symptoms, signs, causes and treatment of corneal disease.
- The difference between episcleritis and scleritis.

Introduction

Disorders of the conjunctiva and cornea are a common cause of symptoms. The ocular surface is regularly exposed to the external environment and subject to trauma, infection and allergic reactions – which account for the majority of diseases in these tissues. Degenerative and structural abnormalities account for a minority of problems.

Symptoms

Patients may complain of the following:

1 Pain and irritation. Conjunctivitis alone is seldom associated with anything more than mild discomfort. Pain signifies something more serious such as corneal injury or infection. This symptom helps differentiate conjunctivitis from corneal disease.

2 Redness. In conjunctivitis the entire conjunctival surface including that covering the tarsal plates is involved. If the redness is localized to the limbus (*a ciliary flush*) the following should be considered:

a keratitis (an inflammation of the cornea);

b uveitis;

c acute glaucoma.

3 Discharge. Purulent discharge suggests a bacterial conjunctivitis. Viral conjunctivitis is associated mainly with a watery discharge.

4 Visual loss which is not cleared by blinking. This occurs only when the central
cornea is affected. Loss of vision is thus an important symptom requiring urgent
action.

5 Patients with corneal disease may also complain of photophobia.

Signs

The following features may be seen in conjunctival disease:

● Papillae. These are raised lesions on the upper tarsal conjunctiva, about 1 mm or
more in diameter with a central vascular core. They are non-specific signs of
chronic inflammation. They result from fibrous septa between the conjunctiva
and subconjunctiva which allow only the intervening tissue to swell with
inflammatory infiltrate. *Giant papillae*, found in allergic eye disease, are formed by
the coalescence of papillae (see Fig. 7.4).

● Follicles (Fig. 7.1). These are raised, gelatinous, oval lesions about 1 mm in diameter, found usually in the lower tarsal conjunctiva and upper tarsal border, and
occasionally at the limbus. Each follicle represents a lymphoid collection with its
own germinal centre. Unlike papillae, the causes of follicles are more specific (e.g.
viral and chlamydial infections).

● Dilation of the conjunctival vasculature (termed *injection*).

● Subconjunctival haemorrhage, often bright red in colour because it is fully oxy-
genated by the ambient air, through the conjunctiva.

The features of corneal disease are different, and include the following:

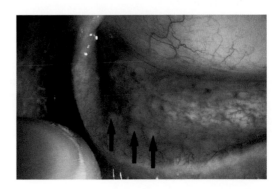

Figure 7.1 The clinical
appearance of follicles.

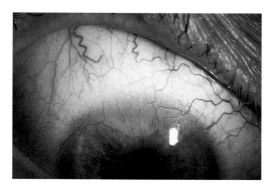

Figure 7.2 Pannus.

- Epithelial and stromal oedema may develop, causing clouding of the cornea.
- Cellular infiltrate in the stroma causing focal granular white spots.
- Deposits of cells on the corneal endothelium (termed *keratic precipitates* or *KPs*, usually lymphocytes or macrophages; see Chapter 9).
- Chronic keratitis may stimulate new blood vessels superficially, under the epithelium (*pannus*; Fig. 7.2) or deeper in the stroma. Stromal oedema, which causes swelling and separates the collagen lamellae, facilitates vessel invasion.
- Epithelial erosions are punctate or more extensive patches of epithelial loss which are best detected using fluorescein dye and viewed with a blue light.

Conjunctiva

Inflammatory diseases of the conjunctiva

Bacterial conjunctivitis

Patients present with:
- redness of the eye;
- discharge;
- ocular irritation.

The commonest causative organisms are *Staphylococcus*, *Streptococcus*, *Pneumococcus* and *Haemophilus*. The condition is usually self-limiting, although a broadspectrum antibiotic eye drop will hasten resolution. Conjunctival swabs for culture are indicated if the condition fails to resolve.

Ophthalmia neonatorum

Ophthalmia neonatorum, which refers to any conjunctivitis that occurs in the first

Antibiotics

Some of the antibiotics available for topical ophthalmic use. Chloramphenicol is an effective broad-spectrum agent; an unproven risk of bone-marrow aplasia is a moot point.
- Ceftazidine
- Chloramphenicol
- Ciprofloxacin
- Fusidic acid
- Gentamicin
- Neomycin
- Tetracycline

28 days of neonatal life, is a notifiable disease. **Swabs for culture are mandatory**. It is also important that the cornea is examined to exclude any ulceration.

The commonest causative agents are:
- Bacterial conjunctivitis (usually Gram-positive).
- *Neisseria gonorrhoeae*. In severe cases this can cause corneal perforation. Penicillin, given topically and systemically, is used to treat local and systemic disease respectively.
- Herpes simplex, which can cause corneal scarring. Topical antivirals are used to treat the condition.
- *Chlamydia*. This may be responsible for a chronic conjunctivitis and cause sight-threatening corneal scarring. Topical tetracycline ointment and systemic erythromycin are used to treat the local and systemic disease respectively.

Viral conjunctivitis

This is distinguished from bacterial conjunctivitis by:
- a watery and limited purulent discharge;
- the presence of conjunctival follicles (hence *follicular conjunctivitis*). Pre-auricular lymph nodes are also enlarged;
- there may also be lid oedema and excessive lacrimation.

The commonest causative agent is adenovirus, and to a much lesser extent Coxsackie and picornavirus. Adenovirus conjunctivitis is self-limiting but highly contagious and frequently occurs in epidemics. There is a risk of hospital-acquired infection, which can arise where there is failure to hand-wash and disinfect equipment. Certain adenovirus serotypes also cause a troublesome punctate keratoconjunctivitis, in which vision is affected, and which may have visual sequelae. Adenoviruses can also cause a conjunctivitis associated with the formation of a pseudomembrane across the conjunctiva. Treatment for the conjunctivitis is unnecessary unless there is a secondary bacterial infection. Patients must be given hygiene instruction to minimize the spread of infection (e.g. using separate towels). Treatment of keratoconjunctivitis is controversial. No effective commercial antiviral is available. The use of topical steroids damps down symptoms and causes corneal opacities to resolve, but rebound inflammation is common when the steroid is stopped, and corneal opacities reappear.

Chlamydial infections

Different serotypes of the obligate intracellular organism *Chlamydia trachomatis* are responsible for two forms of ocular infections.

Inclusion keratoconjunctivitis

This is a sexually transmitted disease and may take a chronic course (up to 18 months) unless adequately treated. Patients present with a mucopurulent follicular conjunctivitis and develop a micropannus (superficial peripheral corneal vascularization and scarring) associated with subepithelial scarring. Urethritis or cervicitis is common. Diagnosis is confirmed by detection of chlamydial antigens, using immunofluorescence, or by identification of typical inclusion bodies by Giemsa staining in conjunctival swab or scrape specimens.

Inclusion conjunctivitis is treated with topical and systemic tetracycline. The patient should be referred to a sexually transmitted diseases clinic.

Trachoma

This is the commonest infective cause of blindness in the world, although it is uncommon in developed countries (more details will be found in Chapter 17). The housefly acts as a vector, and the disease is encouraged by poor hygiene and over-crowding in a dry, hot climate. The hallmark of the disease is subconjunctival fibrosis caused by frequent re-infections associated with the unhygienic conditions. Blindness may occur due to corneal scarring from recurrent keratitis and trichiasis (Fig. 7.3).

Trachoma is treated with oral or topical tetracycline or erythromycin. Azithromycin, an alternative, requires only a single oral dose. Entropion and trichiasis require surgical correction.

Allergic conjunctivitis

This may be divided into acute and chronic forms:

1 Acute (hayfever, or seasonal allergic conjunctivitis) is an acute IgE-mediated reaction to airborne allergens (usually pollens, e.g. ragweed, and mite allergens). Symptoms and signs include:

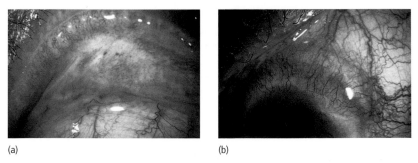

(a)   (b)

Figure 7.3 Trachoma: scarring of (a) the upper lid (everted) and (b) the cornea.

a itchiness;

b conjunctival injection and swelling (chemosis);

c lacrimation.

2 Vernal conjunctivitis (spring catarrh) is also mediated by IgE. It often affects male children with a history of atopy. It is usually seasonal but may be present all year long. Symptoms and signs include:

a itchiness;

b photophobia;

c lacrimation;

d papillary conjunctivitis on the upper tarsal plate (papillae may coalesce to form giant cobblestones; Fig. 7.4);

e limbal follicles and white spots;

f punctate lesions on the corneal epithelium;

g an opaque, oval plaque which in severe disease replaces an upper zone of the corneal epithelium.

Initial therapy is with mast cell stabilizers (e.g. sodium cromoglycate, nedocromil, lodoxamide) or antihistamines (e.g. levocabastine), or with agents combining

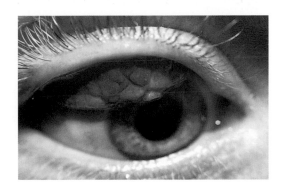

Figure 7.4 The appearance of giant (cobblestone) papillae in vernal conjunctivitis.

mast cell stabilizing and antihistamine properties (e.g. olopatidine). Topical steroids are required in severe cases but long-term use is avoided if possible because of the risks of steroid-induced glaucoma or cataract.

Contact lens wearers may develop an allergic reaction to their lenses or to lens cleaning materials, leading to a *giant papillary conjunctivitis (GPC)* with a mucoid discharge. Whilst this may respond to topical treatment with mast cell stabilizers, it is often necessary to stop lens wear for a period, or even permanently if symptoms recur.

Conjunctival degenerations

Cysts are common in the conjunctiva. They rarely cause symptoms, but if necessary can be removed.

Pingueculae and *pterygia* are found on the interpalpebral bulbar conjunctiva (Fig. 7.5). They are thought to result from excessive exposure to the reflected or direct ultraviolet component of sunlight. Histologically the collagen structure is altered. Pingueculae are small, elevated yellowish paralimbal lesions that never impinge on the cornea. Pterygia are wing-shaped and located nasally, with the apex towards the cornea, onto which they progressively extend. They may cause irritation and, if extensive, may encroach onto the visual axis. They can be excised but may recur.

Conjunctival tumours

These are rare. They include:
• Squamous cell carcinoma. An irregular raised area of conjunctiva which may invade the deeper tissues.
• Malignant melanoma. The differential diagnosis from benign pigmented lesions (for example a naevus) may be difficult. Review is necessary to assess whether the lesion is increasing in size. Biopsy, to achieve a definitive diagnosis, may be required.

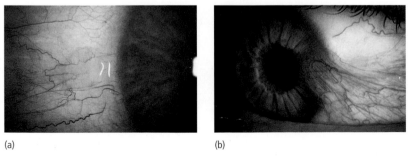

(a)   (b)

Figure 7.5 The clinical appearance of (a) a pinguecula; (b) a pterygium.

Cornea

Infective corneal lesions

Herpes simplex keratitis

Type 1 herpes simplex (HSV) is a common and important cause of ocular disease. Type 2, which causes genital disease, may occasionally cause keratitis and infantile chorioretinitis. Primary infection by HSV1 is usually acquired early in life by close contact such as kissing. It may be asymptomatic, but otherwise is accompanied by:
- fever;
- vesicular lid lesions;
- follicular conjunctivitis;
- pre-auricular lymphadenopathy.

Primary infection may cause a conjunctivitis, with or without punctate keratitis. It is followed by resolution and latency of the virus in the trigeminal ganglion. 'Recurrent' infection involves reactivation of the latent virus, which travels centrifugally to nerve terminals in the corneal epithelium to cause an epithelial keratitis. There may be no past clinical history. The risk of reactivation is increased if the patient is debilitated (e.g. psychiatric disease, systemic illness, immunosuppression). The pathognomonic appearance is of a *dendritic ulcer* (Fig. 7.6). These ulcers may heal without a scar but they may progress to a stromal keratitis, associated with an inflammatory infiltration, and oedema, and ultimately a loss of corneal transparency and permanent scarring. If corneal scarring is severe a corneal graft may be required to restore vision. Uveitis and glaucoma may accompany the disease. *Disciform keratitis* is an immunogenic reaction to herpes antigen in the stroma and presents as stromal oedema and clouding without ulceration, often associated with iritis.

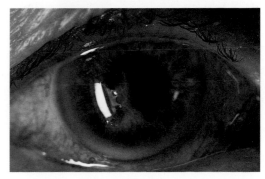

Figure 7.6 A dendritic ulcer seen in herpes simplex infection.

Antivirals

Some of the topical antiviral agents available for ocular therapy:
- Vidarabine
- Trifluorothymidine
- Aciclovir
- Ganciclovir

Dendritic lesions are treated with topical antivirals and typically heal within two weeks. In the UK the standard treatment is with aciclovir. Topical steroids must not be given to patients with a dendritic ulcer, since they may cause extensive corneal ulceration. In patients with stromal involvement (keratitis), steroids are used under ophthalmic supervision and with antiviral cover.

Herpes zoster ophthalmicus (ophthalmic shingles)

This is caused by the varicella zoster virus which is responsible for chickenpox (Fig. 7.7). The ophthalmic division of the trigeminal nerve is affected. Unlike herpes simplex infection, there is usually a prodromal period with the patient systemically unwell. Ocular manifestations are usually preceded by the appearance of vesicles in the distribution of the ophthalmic division of the trigeminal nerve. Ocular problems are more likely if the nasociliary branch of the nerve is involved (signaled by vesicles at the root of the nose). Signs include:

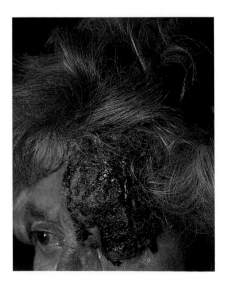

Figure 7.7 The clinical appearance of herpes zoster ophthalmicus.

- lid swelling (which may be bilateral);
- keratitis;
- iritis;
- secondary glaucoma.

Reactivation of the disease is often linked to unrelated systemic illness. Oral antiviral treatment (e.g. aciclovir, famciclovir) is effective in reducing post-infective neuralgia (a severe chronic pain in the area of the rash) if given within three days of the skin vesicles erupting. Ocular disease may require treatment with topical and steroids and antibacterials to cover secondary infection.

The prognosis of herpetic eye disease has improved since antiviral treatment became available. Both simplex and zoster cause anaesthesia of the cornea. Non-healing indolent ulcers may be seen following simplex infection, and these are difficult to treat.

Bacterial keratitis

Bacteria

Some of the bacteria responsible for corneal infection:
- *Staphylococcus epidermidis*
- *Staphylococcus aureus*
- *Streptococcus pneumoniae*
- Coliforms
- *Pseudomonas*
- *Haemophilus*

Pathogenesis

A host of bacteria may infect the cornea. Some are found on the lid margin as part of the normal flora. The conjunctiva and cornea are protected against infection by:
- blinking;
- washing away of debris by the flow of tears;
- entrapment of foreign particles by mucus;
- the antibacterial properties of the tears;
- the barrier function of the corneal epithelium (*Neisseria gonorrhoeae* is the only organism that can penetrate the intact epithelium).

Predisposing causes of bacterial keratitis include:
- keratoconjunctivitis sicca (dry eye);
- a breach in the corneal epithelium (e.g. following trauma);
- contact lens wear;
- prolonged use of topical steroids.

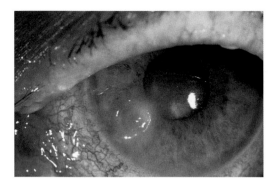

Figure 7.8 Clinical appearance of a corneal ulcer.

Symptoms and signs
These include:
- pain, usually severe unless the cornea is anaesthetic;
- purulent discharge;
- ciliary injection;
- visual loss (severe if the visual axis is involved);
- hypopyon sometimes (a mass of white cells collected in the anterior chamber; see Chapter 9);
- a white corneal opacity which can often be seen with the naked eye (Fig. 7.8).

Treatment
Scrapes are taken from the base of the ulcer for Gram staining and culture. The patient is then treated with intensive topical antibiotics, often with dual therapy using specially formulated, concentrated, combined preparations (e.g. cefuroxime against Gram-positive bacteria and gentamicin for Gram-negative bacteria) to cover most organisms. The use of fluoroquinolones (e.g. ciprofloxacin, ofloxacin, available commercially) as a monotherapy is gaining popularity. The drops are given hourly, day and night, for the first couple of days and reduced in frequency as clinical improvement occurs. In severe or unresponsive disease the cornea may perforate. This can be treated initially with tissue adhesives (cyanoacrylate glue) and a subsequent corneal graft. A persistent scar may also require a corneal graft to restore vision.

Acanthamoeba keratitis
This freshwater amoeba is responsible for infective keratitis (Fig. 7.9). The infection has become more common with the increasing use of soft contact lenses. A painful keratitis with prominent, infiltrated corneal nerves results. The amoeba can be isolated from the cornea (and from the contact lens case) with a scrape and

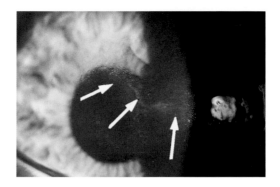

Figure 7.9 The clinical appearance of acanthamoeba keratitis. Arrows indicate neurokeratitis.

cultured on special plates impregnated with *Escherichia coli*. Topical chlorhexidine, polyhexamethylene biguanide (PHMB) and propamidine are used to treat the condition.

Fungal keratitis

This is unusual in the UK but more common in warmer climates such as the southern USA. In India it accounts for 30–50% of infective keratitis. It should be considered in:

- lack of response to antibacterial therapy in corneal ulceration;
- cases of trauma with vegetable matter;
- cases associated with the prolonged use of steroids.

The corneal opacity appears fluffy, and satellite lesions may be present. Liquid and solid Sabouraud's media are used to grow the fungi. Incubation may need to be prolonged. Treatment requires topical antifungal drops such as pimaricin 5%.

Interstitial keratitis

This term is used for any keratitis that affects the corneal stroma without epithelial involvement. Classically the most common cause was congenital syphilis, leaving a midstromal scar interlaced with the empty ('ghost') blood vessels. Corneal grafting may be required when the opacity is marked and visual acuity reduced.

Corneal dystrophies

These are rare inherited disorders. They affect different layers of the cornea and often affect corneal transparency (Fig. 7.10). They may be divided into:

- Anterior dystrophies involving the epithelium. These may present with recurrent corneal erosion.

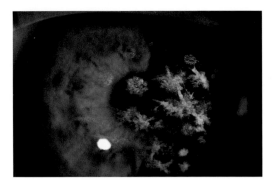

Figure 7.10 Example of a corneal dystrophy (granular dystrophy).

- Stromal dystrophies presenting with visual loss. If very anterior they may cause corneal erosion and pain.
- Posterior dystrophies which affect the endothelium and cause gradual loss of vision due to oedema. They may also cause pain due to epithelial erosion.

Disorders of shape

Keratoconus

This is usually a sporadic disorder but may occasionally be inherited. Thinning of the centre of the cornea leads to an ectatic, conical, corneal shape. Vision is affected but there is no pain. Initially the associated astigmatism can be corrected with glasses or contact lenses. In severe cases a corneal graft may be required.

Central corneal degenerations

Band keratopathy

Band keratopathy is the subepithelial deposition of calcium phosphate in the exposed part of the cornea where CO_2 loss and the consequent raised pH favour its deposition (Fig. 7.11). It is seen in eyes with chronic uveitis or glaucoma, and may cause visual loss or discomfort if epithelial erosions form over the band. If symptomatic it can be scraped off surgically, aided by a chelating agent such as sodium edetate. The excimer laser can also be effective in treating these patients by ablating the affected surface. Band keratopathy can also be a sign of systemic hypercalcaemia, as in hyperparathyroidism or renal failure. The lesion is then more likely to occupy the 3 o'clock and 9 o'clock positions of the paralimbal cornea.

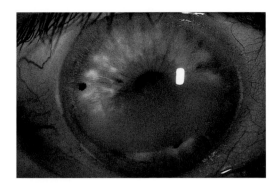

Figure 7.11 Band keratopathy.

Peripheral corneal degenerations

Corneal thinning

A rare cause of painful peripheral corneal thinning is *Mooren's ulcer*, a condition of progressive corneal melting with an immune basis. Corneal melting can also be seen in collagen diseases such as rheumatoid arthritis and Wegener's granulomatosis. Treatment can be difficult, and both sets of disorder require systemic and topical immunosuppression and anti-proteases. Where there is an associated dry eye it is important to ensure adequate corneal wetting and corneal protection (see Chapter 6).

Lipid arcus

This is a peripheral white ring-shaped lipid deposit, separated from the limbus by a clear interval. It is often seen in normal, elderly people (*arcus senilis*), but in younger patients, under 50 years it may be a sign of hyperlipoproteinaemia. No eye treatment is required.

Corneal grafting

Donor corneal tissue can be grafted into a host cornea to restore corneal clarity or repair a perforation (Fig. 7.12). Donor corneas can be stored and are banked so that corneal grafts can be performed on routine operating lists. The avascular host cornea provides an immune-privileged site for grafting, with a high success rate. Tissue can be HLA-typed for grafting of vascularized corneas at high risk of immune rejection, although the value of this is still uncertain. The patient is treated with steroid eye drops for some time after the operation to prevent graft

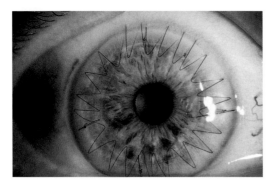

Figure 7.12 A corneal graft. Note the interrupted and the continuous sutures at the interface between graft and host.

rejection. Complications such as astigmatism can be dealt with surgically or by suture adjustment.

Graft rejection

Any patient who has had a corneal graft and who complains of redness, pain or visual loss must be seen urgently by an eye specialist, as this may indicate graft rejection. Examination shows graft oedema, iritis and a line of activated T cells attacking the graft endothelium. Intensive topical steroid application in the early stages can restore graft clarity.

Sclera

Episcleritis

This inflammation of the superficial layer of the sclera causes mild discomfort. It is rarely associated with systemic disease. It is usually self-limiting but, as symptoms are tiresome, topical anti-inflammatory treatment can be given. In rare, severe disease, systemic non-steroidal anti-inflammatory treatment may be helpful.

Scleritis

This is a more severe condition than episcleritis, and may be associated with the collagen vascular diseases, most commonly rheumatoid arthritis. It is a cause of intense ocular pain. Both inflammatory areas and ischaemic areas of the sclera may occur. Characteristically the affected sclera is swollen (Fig. 7.13). The following may complicate the condition:

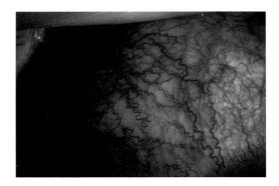

Figure 7.13 The appearance of scleritis.

- scleral thinning (*scleromalacia*), sometimes with perforation;
- keratitis;
- uveitis;
- cataract formation;
- glaucoma.

Treatment may require high doses of systemic steroids, or in severe cases cytotoxic therapy and investigation to find any associated systemic disease.

Scleritis affecting the posterior part of the globe may cause choroidal effusions, or may simulate a tumour.

Key points

- Avoid the unsupervised use of topical steroids in treating ophthalmic conditions, since complications may be serious.
- In contact lens wearers a painful red eye is serious; it may imply an infective keratitis.
- Redness, pain and reduced vision in a patient with corneal graft suggest rejection, which is an ophthalmic emergency.

Multiple choice questions

1. An 11-year-old child presents with a red watery eye and slightly blurred vision. Her sister had similar symptoms a week ago. The appearance of the eye is shown in Fig. 7.14.

a The most likely diagnosis is uveitis.

b The most likely diagnosis is viral conjunctivitis.

c The most likely diagnosis is bacterial conjunctivitis.

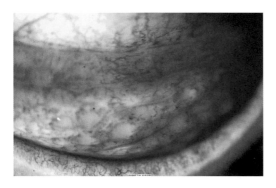

Figure 7.14 The clinical appearance of the eye referred to in Question 1.

d The child should be treated with steroids.

e Papillae are present as elevations on the lid mucosa.

2. A 26-year-old patient presents with an itchy watery eye. She is photophobic and the vision has become blurred. She has a history of asthma. The appearance of the eye is shown in Fig. 7.15.

a The most likely diagnosis is uveitis.

b The most likely diagnosis is epithelial herpes simplex keratitis.

c The most likely diagnosis is allergic conjunctivitis.

d Treatment is with antihistamines, mast cell stabilizers and topical steroids.

e Treatment is with aciclovir.

3. A 67-year-old lady presents with pain on the right side of her forehead. She has been feeling generally unwell. She has just noticed the appearance of vesicles on the skin.

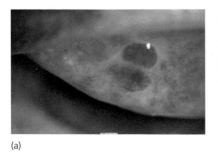 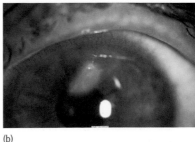

(a)   (b)

Figure 7.15 The clinical appearance of the eye referred to in Question 2.

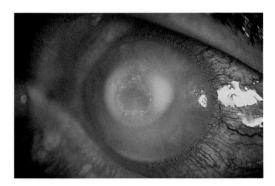

Figure 7.16 The clinical appearance of the eye referred to in Question 4.

a The most likely diagnosis is herpes simplex.
b The most likely diagnosis is herpes zoster.
c The most likely diagnosis is acanthamoeba keratitis.
d Ocular complications may include keratitis, iritis and secondary glaucoma.
e The patient should be prescribed systemic aciclovir in high dosage.

4. A contact lens wearer presents with a red painful eye. There is a purulent discharge and vision is decreased. Figure 7.16 shows the appearance of the eye.
a The most likely diagnosis is a bacterial corneal ulcer.
b Acanthamoeba keratitis is another possibility in a contact lens wearer.
c The most likely diagnosis is a corneal dystrophy.
d The patient has band keratopathy.
e Treatment with intensive topical antibiotics is necessary.

5. A 24-year-old lady presents with a red eye. There is no discharge. The redness is located in the temporal quadrant of the bulbar conjuctiva. There is slight discomfort; the vision is normal. There is no other medical history.
a The most likely diagnosis is bacterial conjunctivitis.
b The most likely diagnosis is keratoconus.
c The most likely diagnosis is episcleritis.
d The most likely diagnosis is scleritis.
e Treatment is with topical steroids or a non-steroidal anti-inflammatory agent.

6. Identify the conditions shown in Fig. 7.17 (a, b and c).

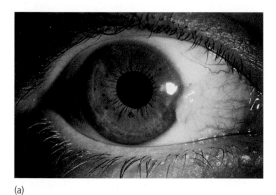

(a)

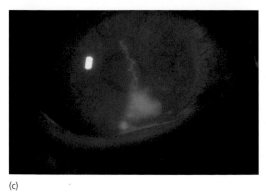

(b)

(c)

Figure 7.17 See Question 6.

Answers

1. An 11-year-old child presents with a red watery eye and slightly blurred vision.

a False. While the symptom of redness fits, the watering and similar symptoms experienced by her sister suggest that an infection is more likely.

b True. The symptoms are typical of an adenovirus conjunctivitis, a condition which is highly contagious.

c False. The discharge would be mucopurulent.

d False. While steroids can help the corneal complications of adenovirus infection, they are difficult to wean. Also, you would wish to exclude a herpes simplex infection before considering their use.

e False. These elevations are called 'follicles' and are composed of lymphoid cells.

2. A 26-year-old patient presents with an itchy watery eye.

a False. The inflammation is not localized at the limbus, papillae are present, and there is an opaque corneal plaque on the cornea.

b False. The corneal lesion does not resemble a dendritic ulcer.

c True. The redness, papillae and corneal lesion are typical of severe vernal keratoconjunctivitis.

d True.

e False. Aciclovir is an antiviral agent used in the treatment of herpes simplex keratitis.

3. A 67-year-old lady presents with pain on the right side of her forehead.

a False. Vesicles would not be a feature of the disease in this age group.

b True.

c False. The skin is not affected in acanthamoeba keratitis.

d True.

e True. If this is given in the first three days of the disease it can reduce symptoms and help prevent severe post-herpetic neuralgia.

4. A contact lens wearer presents with a red painful eye.

a True. Contact lens wear is the commonest risk factor in the developed world. Other causes are trauma, prolonged steroid use, dry eye and an anaesthetic cornea (as seen in herpetic eye disease).

b True. The eye is usually very painful.

c False. These rarely cause a red painful eye.

d False. Band keratopathy is caused by a deposition of calcium salts in the superficial cornea. It may sometimes cause a red painful eye, but the appearance differs.

e True. This is an ophthalmic emergency.

5. A 24-year-old lady presents with a red eye.

a False. There is no discharge and injection is not usually localized in conjunctivitis.

b False. Keratoconus is a disorder of corneal shape and occurs in a white eye.

c True. The symptoms and signs are very suggestive.

d False. The diagnosis is possible but less likely than episcleritis. Scleritis causes a deep, boring pain.

e True. Simple episcleritis is self-limiting. Nodular episcleritis may be helped by topical anti-inflammatory agents. If there is a lack of response, a systemic NSAID (e.g. flurbiprofen) may be used.

6. Identify the conditions shown in Fig. 7.17.

a Pterygium.

b Band keratopathy.

c Herpes simplex dendritic ulcer stained with fluorescein.

Chapter 8

The lens and cataract

Learning objectives

To understand:
- The pathology of cataract; its symptoms, signs and causes.
- The reasons for undertaking cataract surgery.
- The principles of the different forms of cataract surgery.
- The complications of cataract surgery.

Introduction

The lens is biconvex and transparent and is held in position behind the iris by the suspensory ligament, whose zonular fibres are composed of the protein fibrillin and attach the equator of the lens to the ciliary body. Disease may affect structure, shape and position.

Change in lens structure

Cataract

Opacification of the lens of the eye (*cataract*) is the commonest cause of treatable blindness in the world. The large majority of cataracts occur in older subjects, as a result of cumulative exposure to environmental and other influences such as smoking, UV radiation and elevated blood sugar levels. This is sometimes referred to as *age-related cataract*. Age of onset is lower in countries with the highest prevalence of cataract. A smaller number are associated with specific ocular or systemic

---

Ocular conditions associated with cataract

- Trauma
- Uveitis
- High myopia
- Topical medication (particularly steroid eye drops)
- Intraocular tumour

---

disease and defined physicochemical mechanisms. Some are congenital and may be inherited.

Symptoms

An opacity in the lens of the eye:
- causes a painless loss of vision;
- causes glare;
- may change refractive error.

In infants, cataract may cause *amblyopia* (a failure of normal visual development) because the retina is deprived of a formed image. Infants with suspected cataract or a family history of congenital cataracts should be assessed by an ophthalmologist shortly after birth, as a matter of urgency (see *Congenital cataract*, below).

Signs

Visual acuity is reduced. In some patients the acuity, measured in a dark room, may seem satisfactory, but if the same test is carried out in bright light or sunlight the acuity falls, as a result of glare and loss of contrast. Also the smaller pupils may restrict light entry.

A cataract appears black against the red reflex when the eye is examined with a direct ophthalmoscope (see Chapter 2). Slit lamp examination allows the cataract

---

Systemic causes of cataract

- Diabetes
- Other metabolic disorders (including galactosaemia, Fabry disease, hypocalcaemia)
- Systemic drugs (particularly steroids, chlorpromazine)
- Infection (congenital rubella)
- Myotonic dystrophy
- Atopic dermatitis
- Systemic syndromes (Down's, Lowe's)
- Congenital, including inherited, cataract
- X-radiation

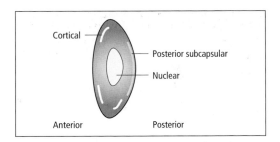

Figure 8.1 The location of different types of cataract.

to be examined in detail, and the exact site of the opacity in the lens can be identified. Age-related cataract is commonly nuclear, cortical or subcapsular in location (Fig. 8.1). Steroid-induced cataract is commonly posterior subcapsular. Other features to suggest an ocular cause for the cataract may be found, for example pigment deposition on the lens suggesting previous inflammation, or damage to the iris suggesting previous ocular trauma (Fig. 8.2).

Investigation

This is seldom required, unless a suspected systemic disease requires exclusion or the cataract appears to have occurred at an early age.

Treatment

Although much effort has been directed towards slowing progression or preventing cataract, management remains surgical. There is no need to wait for the cataract to 'ripen' and cause major visual loss. The test is whether or not the cataract produces sufficient visual symptoms to reduce the quality of life. Patients may have difficulty in recognizing faces, reading, carrying out their occupation or achieving the driving standard. Some patients may be greatly troubled by glare. Prior to surgery patients must be informed of any coexisting eye disease which may influence the outcome of cataract surgery and the visual prognosis.

Cataract surgery

The operation (Fig. 8.3) involves gaining access to the lens substance via a hole made in the anterior part of the lens capsule, removal of most of the lens fibres and epithelial cells, and insertion of a plastic lens implant of appropriate optical power. The implant is held in place within the 'capsular bag' and the thin, transparent posterior capsule offers no obstruction to light entering the eye.

Surgery is increasingly performed under local rather than general anaesthesia. Local anaesthetic is infiltrated around the globe and the lids or given topically. If

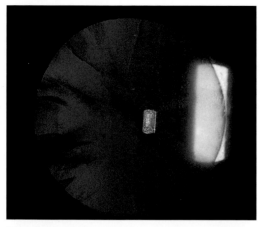

(a)

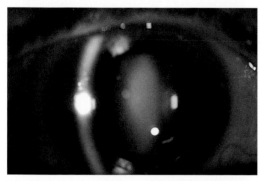

(b)

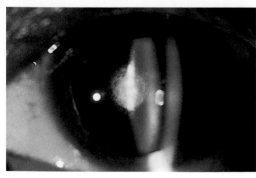

(c)

Figure 8.2 The clinical appearance of (a) a cortical, (b) a nuclear, (c) a posterior subcapsular cataract. The spoke opacities are silhouetted against the red reflex in (a).

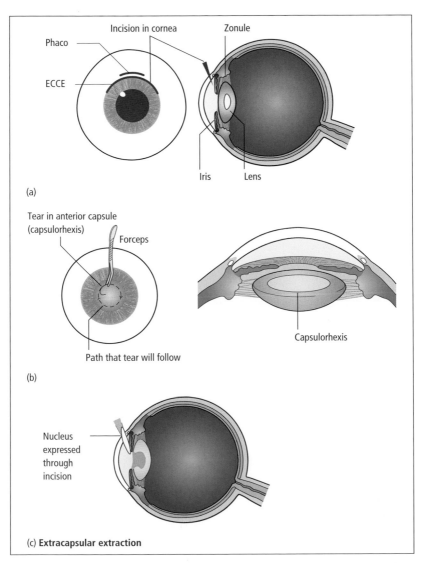

Figure 8.3 Stages in the removal of a cataract and the placement of an intraocular lens. (a) An incision is made in the cornea or anterior sclera. A small, stepped self-sealing incision is made for phacoemulsification. (b) A circular disc of the anterior capsule is removed. A variety of different methods are used to do this. In ECCE a ring of small incisions is made with a needle to perforate the capsule, allowing the central portion to be removed. In phacoemulsification the capsule is torn in a circle leaving a strong smooth edge to the remaining anterior capsule. A cannula is then placed under the anterior capsule and fluid injected to separate the lens nucleus from the cortex, allowing the nucleus to be rotated within the capsular bag. (c) In ECCE the hard nucleus of the lens is removed through the incision, by *expression*. Pressure on the eye causes the nucleus to pass out through the incision.

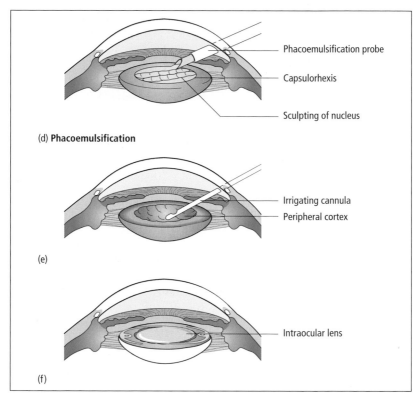

(d) Phacoemulsification

Phacoemulsification probe

Capsulorhexis

Sculpting of nucleus

(e)

Irrigating cannula
Peripheral cortex

(f)

Intraocular lens

Figure 8.3 (*continued*) (d) Alternatively the nucleus can be emulsified *in situ*. The phacoemulsification probe, introduced through the small corneal or scleral incision, shaves away the nucleus. (e) The remaining soft lens matter is aspirated, leaving only the posterior capsule and the peripheral part of the anterior capsule. (f) An intraocular lens is implanted into the remains of the capsule. To allow implantation through the small phacoemulsification wound, the lens must be folded in half or injected through a special introducer into the eye. The incision is repaired with fine nylon sutures. If phacoemulsification has been used the incision in the eye is smaller and a suture is usually not required.

social circumstances allow, the patient can attend as a day case, without admission to hospital.

The operation can be performed:

• Through an extended incision at the limbus, followed by *extracapsular cataract extraction (ECCE)* (Fig. 8.3c). Here, the bulk of the lens substance is expressed from the eye with gentle pressure and residual material aspirated with a cannula. The incision must be sutured and the sutures removed post operatively.

• By liquefication of the lens using an ultrasound probe introduced through a smaller incision at the limbus (*phacoemulsification*) (Fig. 8.3d). Usually no suture is required. This is now the preferred method in the Western world.

The optical power of the *lens implant* is calculated prior to surgery by measuring the length of the eye ultrasonically and the curvature of the cornea (and thus its optical power) optically. The power of the lens is generally calculated to provide good distance acuity without glasses (i.e. emmetropia). The choice of implant power is influenced by the refraction of the fellow eye and whether it too has a cataract which will require surgery. Where surgery on the fellow eye is likely to be delayed, it is important that the patient is not left with a major difference in the refractive state of the two eyes (aniseikonia), since the difference in retinal image size may not be tolerated visually.

Postoperatively the patient is given a short course of steroid and antibiotic drops. New glasses can be prescribed after a few weeks, once the incision has healed. Visual rehabilitation and the prescription of new glasses is much quicker after phacoemulsification. Since the patient cannot accommodate, a spectacle correction will be required postoperatively for close work even if it is not needed for distance. Multifocal intraocular lenses, which provide good distance and near vision without glasses, are now in use, although there may be a reduction in contrast sensitivity with these lenses. Accommodating intraocular lenses are being developed.

Surgery may sometimes induce a degree of corneal astigmatism. Where sutures were used their post operative removal may reduce this. This is done prior to measuring the patient for new glasses but after the wound has healed and steroid drops have been stopped. Excessive corneal curvature can be induced in the line of a tight suture. Removal usually solves this problem, and is easily accomplished in the clinic under local anaesthetic with the patient sitting at the slit lamp. Loose sutures must be removed to prevent infection but it may be necessary to resuture the incision if healing is imperfect. Sutureless phacoemulsification through a smaller incision avoids these complications. Furthermore, a modified entry site may allow correction of pre-existing astigmatism.

Complications of cataract surgery

1 Vitreous loss. If the posterior capsule is damaged during the operation the vitreous gel may come forward into the anterior chamber, where it represents a risk for glaucoma or may cause retinal traction. The gel requires careful aspiration and excision (*vitrectomy* at the time of surgery), and placement of the intraocular lens may need to be deferred to a secondary procedure.

2 Iris prolapse. The iris may protrude through the surgical incision in the immediate postoperative period. It appears as a dark area at the incision site. The pupil is distorted. This requires prompt surgical repair.

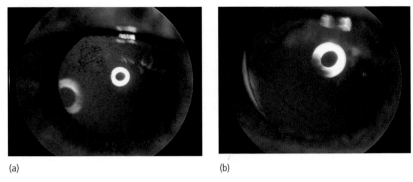

(a)   (b)

Figure 8.4 (a) An opacified posterior capsule. (b) The result of laser capsulotomy.

3 Endophthalmitis. A serious but rare infective complication of cataract extraction (less than 0.3%). Patients present, usually within a few days of surgery, with:
  a a painful red eye;
  b reduced visual acuity;
  c a collection of white cells in the anterior chamber (hypopyon).
The patient requires urgent ophthalmic assessment, sampling of aqueous and vitreous for microbiological analysis, and treatment with intravitreal, topical and systemic antibiotics.
4 Cystoid macular oedema. The macula may become oedematous following surgery, particularly if this has been accompanied by a loss of vitreous. It may settle with time but can produce a severe reduction in acuity. Inflammatory prostaglandin release may play a part in this, and prompt treatment with topical NSAIDs and steroid can alleviate the oedema in a proportion of patients.
5 Retinal detachment. Modern techniques of cataract extraction are associated with a low rate of this complication. It is increased if there has been vitreous loss. The symptoms, signs and management are described in Chapter 11.
6 Opacification of the posterior capsule (Fig. 8.4). In approximately 20% of patients clarity of the posterior capsule decreases in the months following surgery when residual epithelial cells migrate across its surface leading to an opaque scar. Vision becomes blurred and there may be problems with glare. A small hole can be made in the capsule with a laser (*neodymium yttrium garnet (ndYAG) laser*) as an outpatient procedure. There is a small risk of cystoid macular oedema or retinal detachment following YAG capsulotomy. Research aimed at reducing this complication has shown that the lens implant material, the shape of the edge of the lens and overlap of the intraocular lens by a small rim of anterior capsule are important in preventing posterior capsule opacification.

7 If the fine nylon sutures are not removed after surgery they may break in the following months or years, causing irritation or infection. Symptoms are cured by removal.

Congenital cataract

The presence of congenital or infantile cataract is a threat to sight, not only because of the immediate obstruction to vision but because disturbance of the retinal image impairs visual maturation in the infant and leads to amblyopia (see Chapter 15). If bilateral cataract is present and has a significant effect on retinal image formation this will cause amblyopia and an oscillation of the eyes (*nystagmus*). Both cataractous lenses require urgent surgery and the fitting of contact lenses to correct the aphakia. The management of contact lenses requires considerable input and motivation from the parents of the child.

The treatment of uniocular congenital cataract remains controversial. Unfortunately the results of surgery are disappointing and vision may improve little because amblyopia develops despite adequate optical correction with a contact lens. To maximize the chances of success, treatment must be performed within the first few weeks of life and be accompanied by a coordinated patching routine to the fellow eye to stimulate visual maturation in the amblyopic eye. Increasingly, intraocular lenses are being implanted in children over 2 years old. The eye becomes increasingly myopic as the child grows, however, making the choice of lens implant power difficult.

Change in lens shape

Abnormal lens shape is very unusual. The curvature of the anterior part of the lens may be increased centrally (*anterior lenticonus*) in Alport's syndrome, a recessively inherited condition of deafness and nephropathy. An abnormally small lens may be associated with short stature and other skeletal abnormalities.

Change in lens position (ectopia lentis)

Weakness of the zonule causes lens displacement. The lens takes up a more rounded form and the eye becomes more myopic. This may be seen in:
- Trauma.
- Inborn errors of metabolism (e.g. homocystinuria, a recessive disorder with mental defect and skeletal features. The lens is usually displaced downwards).
- Certain syndromes (e.g. Marfan syndrome, a dominant disorder with skeletal and cardiac abnormalities and a risk of dissecting aortic aneurysm. The lens is

usually displaced upwards). There is a defect in the zonular protein due to a mutation in the *fibrillin* gene.

The irregular myopia can be corrected optically, although sometimes an aphakic correction may be required if the lens is substantially displaced from the visual axis. Surgical removal may be indicated, particularly if the displaced lens has caused a secondary glaucoma, but surgery may result in further complications.

Cataract – the world perspective

In the developed world cataract surgery is performed when visual symptoms interfere with the quality of life. Worldwide there are in excess of 20 million people blind due to dense bilateral cataract (for more detail see Chapter 17). This represents a huge cause of preventable blindness. Cataract is a major focus of the Vision 2020 project, a joint initiative of the World Health Organization and the International Association for the Blind. The goal is to remove cataract as a cause of blindness by the year 2020.

Key points

- In adult cataract, extraction is indicated if the reduction in vision is interfering with the patient's quality of life.
- An infant with a family history of congenital cataract or a suspected cataract must be seen by an ophthalmologist as a matter of urgency.

Multiple choice questions

1. Cataract causes:
a A sudden loss of vision.
b A gradual loss of vision.
c Glare.
d Photophobia.
e A change in refractive error.

2. Cataract may be caused by or associated with:
a Trauma.
b Steroids.
c Diabetes.
d Myotonic dystrophy.
e Hypocalcaemia.

3. Complications of cataract surgery include:
a Recurrence of the cataract.
b Endophthalmitis.
c Astigmatism.
d Glaucoma.
e Cystoid macular oedema.

4. A 60-year-old lady has just had a cataract operation. Three days later she presents to her general practitioner with a painful red eye. The vision, which was initially much improved, has become blurred and she is seeing lots of floaters.
a The GP should reassure her that the eye is settling down.
b The patient has endophthalmitis and needs to be referred to an eye unit immediately.
c Treatment of the condition requires steroid drops only.
d Treatment of the condition requires intravitreal antibiotics.
e This is a rare complication of cataract surgery.

Answers

1. Cataract causes:
a False. The change in vision is gradual.
b True.
c True.
d False.
e True. For example, in nuclear cataract an increase in the density of lens proteins at the centre of the lens causes a myopic shift.

2. Cataract may be caused by or associated with:
a True.
b True.
c True.
d True.
e True.

3. Complications of cataract surgery include:
a False. Most lens material is removed by surgery, the cataract does not recur but the posterior capsule may opacify later. Laser capsulotomy can restore vision by creating a hole in the capsule, on the visual axis.
b True.
c True.

d True.
e True.

4. A 60-year-old lady has just had a cataract operation.

a False. The patient has endophthalmitis, a serious eye emergency, and must be referred immediately.

b True.

c False. But these may form part of the treatment in conjunction with antibiotics.

d True.

e True.

Chapter 9

Uveitis

Learning objectives

To understand:
- The definition of uveitis and the ocular structures involved.
- The symptoms, signs, causes and treatment of uveitis.

Introduction

Inflammation of the uveal tract (the iris, ciliary body and choroid) has many causes and is termed *uveitis* (Fig. 9.1). It is usual for structures adjacent to the inflamed uveal tissue to become involved in the inflammatory process. It may be classified anatomically:

- Inflammation of the iris, accompanied by increased vascular permeability, is termed *iritis* or *anterior uveitis* (Fig. 9.2). White cells circulating in the aqueous

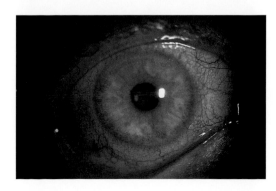

Figure 9.1 External ocular appearance in a patient with uveitis. Note the inflammatory response at the limbus.

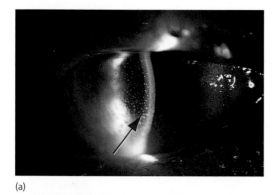

(a)

(b)

(c)

Figure 9.2 Signs of anterior uveitis: (a) keratic precipitates on the corneal endothelium; (b) posterior synechiae (adhesions between the lens and iris) give the pupil an irregular appearance; (c) a hypopyon, white cells collected to form a fluid level in the inferior anterior chamber.

humour of the anterior chamber can be seen with a slit lamp. Protein, which also leaks from the blood vessels, is picked out by its light-scattering properties in the beam of the slit lamp as a '*flare*'.

- An inflammation of the ciliary body is termed *cyclitis*, and of the pars plana, *intermediate uveitis*.
- Inflammation of the posterior uvea, i.e. the choroid (*posterior uveitis* or *choroiditis*), results in inflammatory cells in the vitreous gel. There may also be an associated retinal inflammation (*retinitis*). A *panuveitis* is present when anterior and posterior uveitis occur together.

Epidemiology

The incidence of uveitis is about 15 per 100 000 people. About 75% of these are anterior uveitis.

About 50% of patients with uveitis have an associated systemic disease.

History

The patient may complain of:
- ocular pain (less frequent with posterior uveitis or choroiditis);
- photophobia;
- blurring of vision;
- redness of the eye.

Posterior uveitis may, however, not be painful.

The patient must be questioned about other relevant symptoms that may help determine whether or not there is an associated systemic disease:

- Respiratory symptoms such as shortness of breath, cough, and the nature of any sputum produced (associated sarcoidosis or tuberculosis).
- Skin problems. Erythema nodosum (painful raised red lesions on the arms and shins) may be present in granulomatous diseases such as sarcoidosis and Behçet's disease. Patients with Behçet's may also have thrombophlebitis, dermatographia and oral and genital ulceration. Psoriasis (in association with arthritis) may be accompanied by uveitis.
- Joint disease. Ankylosing spondylitis with back pain is associated with acute anterior uveitis. In children juvenile chronic arthritis may be associated with uveitis. Reiter's disease (classically urethritis, conjunctivitis and a seronegative arthritis) may also be associated with anterior uveitis.
- Bowel disease. Occasionally uveitis may be associated with inflammatory bowel diseases such as ulcerative colitis, Crohn's disease and Whipple's disease.
- Infectious disease. Syphilis with its protean manifestations can cause uveitis (particularly posterior choroiditis). Herpetic disease (shingles) may also cause

uveitis. Cytomegalovirus (CMV) may cause uveitis, particularly in patients with AIDS. Fungal infections and metastatic infections may also cause uveitis, usually in immunocompromised patients.

Signs

On examination:
- The visual acuity may be reduced.
- The eye will be inflamed in acute anterior disease, mostly around the limbus (*ciliary injection*).
- Inflammatory cells may be visible clumped together on the endothelium of the cornea, particularly inferiorly (*keratitic precipitates* or *KPs*).
- Slit-lamp examination will reveal aqueous cells and a flare due to exuded protein. If the inflammation is severe there may be sufficient white cells to collect as a fluid level inferiorly (*hypopyon*).
- The vessels on the iris may be dilated.
- The iris may adhere to the lens and bind down the pupil (*posterior synechiae* or *PS*). Peripheral anterior synechiae (PAS) between the iris and the trabecular meshwork or cornea may occlude the drainage angle.
- The intraocular pressure may be elevated by PAS or increased aqueous protein.
- There may be cells in the vitreous.
- There may be retinal or choroidal foci of inflammation.
- Macular oedema may be present (see Chapter 11).

Investigations

These are aimed at determining a systemic association and are directed in part by the type of uveitis present. An anterior uveitis is more likely to be associated with ankylosing spondylitis, and HLA typing may help confirm the diagnosis. The presence of large KPs and possibly nodules on the iris may suggest sarcoidosis: a chest radiograph, serum calcium and serum angiotensin-converting enzyme levels would be appropriate. In toxoplasmic retinochoroiditis the focus of inflammation often occurs at the margin of an old inflammatory choroidal scar. A posterior uveitis may have an infectious or systemic inflammatory cause. Some diseases such as CMV infections in HIV-positive patients have a characteristic appearance, and with an appropriate history may require no further diagnostic tests. Associated symptoms may also point towards a systemic disease (e.g. fever, diarrhoea, weight loss). Not all cases of anterior uveitis require investigation at first presentation unless associated systemic symptoms are present.

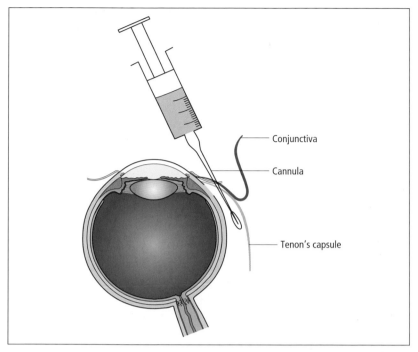

Conjunctiva

Cannula

Tenon's capsule

Figure 9.3 The principle of a sub-Tenon's injection. A cannula is placed in the potential space between the sclera and Tenon's capsule. Injection of steroid separates the two layers and the steroid surrounds the eye.

Treatment

This is aimed at:
- relieving pain and inflammation in the eye;
- preventing damage to ocular structures, particularly to the macula and the optic nerve, which may lead to permanent visual loss.

Steroid therapy is the mainstay of treatment. In anterior uveitis this is delivered by eye drops. However, topical steroids do not effectively penetrate to the posterior segment. Posterior uveitis is therefore treated with systemic steroids, or with steroids injected onto the orbital floor or into the sub-Tenon's space (Fig. 9.3).

In anterior uveitis, dilating the pupil relieves the pain from ciliary spasm and prevents the formation of posterior synechiae by separating it from the anterior lens capsule. Synechiae otherwise interfere with normal dilation of the pupil.

Table 9.1 Some causes of uveitis (not an exhaustive list).

Infectious	Associated with systemic disease	Ocular disease
Toxoplasmosis	Ankylosing spondylosis	Advanced cataract
Postoperative infection	Sarcoidosis	Sympathetic ophthalmitis
Fungal	Reiter's disease	Retinal detachment
CMV	Behçet's disease	Angle closure glaucoma
Herpetic	Psoriatic arthritis	Intraocular tumours
Tuberculosis	Juvenile chronic arthritis	
Syphilis	Inflammatory bowel disease	
Metastatic infection		
Toxocara		

Dilation is achieved with mydriatics, e.g. cyclopentolate or atropine drops. Atropine has a prolonged action lasting weeks. An attempt to break any synechiae that have formed should be made with initial intensive cyclopentolate and phenylephrine drops. A subconjunctival injection of mydriatics may help to break resistant synechiae.

In posterior uveitis/retinitis visual loss may occur either from destructive processes caused by the retinitis itself (e.g. in toxoplasma or CMV) or from fluid accumulation in the layers of the macula (macular oedema). Apart from systemic or injected steroids, specific antiviral or antibiotic medication may also be required. Some rare but severe forms of uveitis, e.g. that associated with Behçet's disease, may require treatment with other systemic immunosuppressive drugs such as azathoprine or cyclosporin. Long-term treatment may be necessary.

Specific conditions associated with uveitis

There are a large number of systemic diseases associated with uveitis. A few of the more common ones are outlined in Table 9.1.

Ankylosing spondylitis

This is a seronegative (rheumatoid factor negative) inflammatory arthritis of the spine. Genetic factors are involved in the disease. Ninety per cent of patients with uveitis have the tissue type HLA B27, although the prevalence of the disease in people in general with HLA B27 is only 1%. Approximately 20% of patients with ankylosing spondylitis will develop acute anterior uveitis. Males are affected more frequently than females (3 : 1).

History

Recurrent anterior uveitis may be the presenting feature of this condition. Close enquiry will usually reveal a history of backache, typically worse on waking and relieved by exercise. Stiffness at rest is a useful symptom which helps differentiate the condition from disease of the intervertebral discs. The peripheral joints may be affected in a minority of patients.

Signs

These are typical of an anterior uveitis.

Investigation

The presence of symptoms and signs in an HLA B27-positive individual is indicative. Sacroiliac spinal X-rays may reveal the classical features of the disease.

Treatment

Ocular treatment is as previously outlined. The patient will benefit from a rheumatological opinion and may require intermittent anti-inflammatory treatment and physiotherapy.

Prognosis

Patients may experience recurrent attacks. The outlook for vision is good if the acute attacks are treated early and vigorously.

Reiter's disease

This condition predominantly affects males, nearly all of whom are HLA B27-positive. It comprises:
- urethritis;
- arthritis (typically of the large joints);
- conjunctivitis.

Some 40% of patients develop acute anterior uveitis.

Juvenile chronic arthritis

A seronegative arthritis (negative for rheumatoid factor) which presents in children, either as a systemic disease with fevers and lymphadenopathy, or as a pauciarticular or polyarticular arthritis. The pauciarticular form has the higher risk of chronic anterior uveitis, particularly if the patient is positive for antinuclear antibodies.

History

The anterior uveitis is chronic and usually asymptomatic. A profound visual defect may be discovered by chance if lens or retinal damage caused by chronic uveitis has developed slowly.

Signs

The eye is white (unusual for iritis), but other signs of an anterior uveitis are present. Because the uveitis is chronic, cataract may occur and patients may develop glaucoma, either as a result of the uveitis or as a result of the steroid drops used to treat the condition. Macular oedema may also occur. Approximately 70% of cases show bilateral involvement.

Investigation

Rheumatoid factor is negative but patients frequently have a positive antinuclear antibody.

Treatment

Ocular treatment is as previously outlined. Patients may be put on systemic treatment for the joint disease. It is important to screen children with juvenile arthritis regularly for uveitis, as they are otherwise asymptomatic unless potentially blinding complications occur. Glaucoma can be very difficult to treat, and if medical treatment fails to control pressure, it may require surgery.

Fuchs' heterochromic uveitis

This is a rare chronic uveitis usually found in young adults. The cause is uncertain, it may be immune mediated and there are no systemic associations.

History

The patient does not usually present with a typical history of iritis. Blurred vision and floaters may be the initial complaint.

Signs

A mild anterior uveitis is present, but without signs of conjunctival inflammation, and there are no posterior synechiae. There are KPs distributed diffusely over the cornea. The iris is heterochromic due to loss of some of the pigment epithelial cells. The vitreous may be inflamed and condensations (the cause of the floaters) may be present. About 70% of patients develop cataract. Glaucoma occurs to a lesser extent.

Treatment

Steroids are not effective in controlling the inflammation and are thus not prescribed. Patients usually respond well to cataract surgery when it is required. The glaucoma is treated conventionally.

Toxoplasmosis

History

The infection may be congenital or acquired. Most ocular toxoplasmosis was thought to be congenital, with the resulting retinochoroiditis being reactivated in adult life. However, there is now evidence that it is often acquired during a glandular fever-like illness. The patient may complain of hazy vision and floaters, and the eye may be red and painful.

Signs

The retina is the principal structure involved, with secondary inflammation occurring in the choroid (*retinochoroiditis*). An active lesion is often located at the posterior pole, appearing as a creamy focus of inflammatory cells at the margin of an old chorioretinal scar (such scars are usually atrophic, with a pigmented edge) (Fig. 9.4). Inflammatory cells cause a vitreous haze, and the anterior chamber may also show evidence of inflammation.

Investigation

The clinical appearance is usually diagnostic, but a positive toxoplasma antibody test is suggestive. However, a high percentage of the population have positive IgG titres due to prior infection.

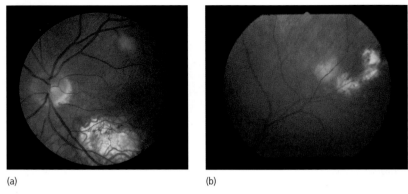

(a)   (b)

Figure 9.4 The appearance of (a) an inactive toxoplasma retinitis and (b) a reactivated lesion. The active lesion appears pale with indistinct edges; it lies above the inactive one.

Treatment

Reactivated lesions will subside, but treatment is required if the macula or optic nerve is threatened or if the inflammatory response is very severe. Systemic steroids are administered with an antiprotozoal drug such as clindamycin. Care must be taken with the use of sulphadiazines or clindamycin, as pseudomembranous colitis may result from clindamycin treatment. Patients must be warned that if diarrhoea develops they should seek medical help immediately.

Acquired immunodeficiency syndrome (AIDS) and CMV retinitis

Ocular disease is a common manifestation of the acquired immunodeficiency syndrome. Patients develop a variety of ocular conditions:
• Microvascular occlusion causing retinal haemorrhages and cotton-wool spots (axonal swelling proximal to infarcted areas of the retinal nerve fibre layer).
• Corneal endothelial deposits.
• Neoplasms of the eye and orbit.
• Neuro-ophthalmic disorders including oculomotor palsies.
• Opportunistic infections, of which the most common is CMV retinitis (previously seen in more than one-third of AIDS patients, but the population at risk has decreased significantly since the advent of highly active anti-retroviral therapy (HAART) in the treatment of AIDS). It typically occurs in patients with a blood CD4+ cell count of less than 50/ml. Toxoplasmosis, herpes simplex and herpes zoster are among other infections that may be seen.

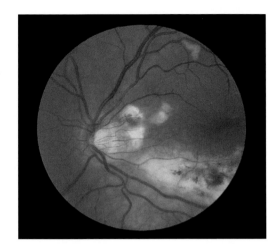

Figure 9.5 The retinal appearance in a patient with AIDS and CMV retinitis. Note the cotton-wool spot at one o'clock.

History

The patient may complain of blurred vision or floaters. A diagnosis of HIV disease has usually already been made and other AIDS-defining features may have presented.

Signs

CMV retinopathy comprises a whitish area of retina, associated with haemorrhage, which has been likened in appearance to 'cottage cheese' (Fig. 9.5). The lesions may threaten the macula or the optic disc. There is usually an associated sparse inflammation of the vitreous.

Treatment

Chronic therapy with ganciclovir and/or foscarnet given parenterally is the current mainstay of therapy; these drugs may also be given *into* the vitreous cavity. Cidofivir is available for intravenous administration. Ganciclovir and its prodrug valganciclovir are available orally. Depot systems for the long-term delivery of anti-CMV agents into the vitreous are under active development, and a ganciclovir implant is available.

Prognosis

Prolonged treatment is required to prevent recurrence.

Sympathetic ophthalmitis

This is a devastating complication of ocular injury. A penetrating or surgical injury to one eye involving the retina may rarely excite a peculiar form of uveitis which involves not only the injured eye but also the fellow eye. This is termed sympathetic ophthalmitis. The uveitis may be so severe that in the worst cases sight may be lost from both eyes. Fortunately systemic steroids, and particularly cyclosporin, have greatly improved the chances of conserving vision. Sympathetic ophthalmitis usually develops within three months of the injury or last ocular operation but may occur at any time. The cause appears to be an immune response against retinal antigens at the time of injury. It can be prevented by enucleation (removal) of the traumatized eye shortly after the injury (within a week or so) if the prospects for visual potential in that eye are very poor and there is major disorganization. Excision must precede the onset of signs in the fellow eye.

Symptoms

The patient may complain of pain and decreased vision in the uninjured fellow eye.

Signs

The iris appears swollen, and yellow-white spots may be seen on the retina. There is a panuveitis.

Treatment

High-dose systemic and topical steroids, and also oral cyclosporin, are required to reduce the inflammation and try to prevent long-term visual loss. It is vital to warn patients with ocular trauma or multiple eye operations to attend an eye casualty department if they experience any problems with their normal eye.

Key points

- Angle closure glaucoma may cause an anterior uveitis and may present with similar symptoms. Look for a dilated pupil and check the intraocular pressure.
- Patients with a retinal detachment may occasionally present with an anterior uveitis. The retina should always be examined in patients with uveitis.
- Active treatment of uveitis is required to prevent long-term complications.
- Children with juvenile arthritis require regular screening to exclude the presence of uveitis, as it is usually asymptomatic.

Multiple Choice Questions

1. Uveitis can be an inflammation of
a The lens.

b The iris.

c The ciliary body.

d The choroid.

e The optic nerve.

2. Uveitis
a Is always associated with a red eye.

b May be complicated by macular oedema.

c Posterior synechiae may form between the iris and the lens.

d May cause oculomotor palsies.

e May be associated with retinitis.

3. A 33-year-old West Indian patient presents with a red eye, without discharge, and with photophobia and blurred vision. The eye is uncomfortable. He has recently become short of breath and developed painful, raised, tender red lesions on his shins.
a The patient has uveitis.

b The patient has ankylosing spondylitis.

c The patient probably has sarcoidosis.

d Treatment is with steroid eye drops and cycloplegics.

e Glaucoma and cataract are possible ocular complications of the condition or its treatment.

4. In acquired immunodeficiency syndrome
a Haemorrhages and cotton-wool spots may be seen on the retina.

b Opportunistic infection has increased since the development of highly active anti-retroviral therapy (HAART).

c CMV retinopathy causes focal white spots on the retina associated with haemorrhage.

d Ganciclovir and foscarnet are used to treat CMV retinitis.

e Oculomotor palsies may be seen in AIDS.

Answers

1. Uveitis can be an inflammation of
a False.

b True.

c True.
d True.
e False.

2. Uveitis
a False. The eye is usually white in children with uveitis associated with juvenile arthritis.
b True.
c True.
d False. The condition affects the eye alone.
e True.

3. A 33-year-old West Indian patient presents with a red eye, without discharge, and with photophobia and blurred vision.
a True. The signs are classical.
b False. Although kyphosis in ankylosing spondylitis may cause shortness of breath, this condition is not associated with erythema nodosum.
c True. The uveitis, shortness of breath and erythema nodosum are suggestive.
d True. And his systemic disease also requires investigation and treatment.
e True. Both anterior uveitis and prolonged treatment with topical steroids my cause cataract or open angle glaucoma. Anterior uveitis may also cause closed angle glaucoma.

4. In acquired immunodeficiency syndrome
a True.
b False. There has been a reduction in opportunistic infection.
c True.
d True.
e True.

Chapter 10

Glaucoma

Learning objectives

To understand.
- The nature of glaucoma.
- The difference between primary and secondary glaucoma; open and closed angle glaucoma.
- The different symptoms and signs of open and closed angle glaucoma.
- The three major forms of glaucoma therapy.

Introduction

The glaucomas comprise a group of diseases in which damage to the optic nerve (optic neuropathy) is usually caused by the effects of raised ocular pressure acting at the optic nerve head. Independent ischaemia of the optic nerve head may also be important. Axon loss results in visual field defects and a loss of visual acuity if the central visual field is involved.

Basic physiology

The intraocular pressure level depends on the balance between production and removal of aqueous humour (Fig. 10.1). Aqueous is produced by secretion and ultrafiltration from the ciliary processes into the posterior chamber. It then passes through the pupil into the anterior chamber, to leave the eye predominantly via the trabecular meshwork, Schlemm's canal and the episcleral veins (*the conventional pathway*). A small proportion of the aqueous (4%) drains across the ciliary body into the supra-choroidal space and into the venous circulation across the sclera (*uveoscleral pathway*).

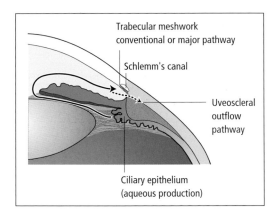

Trabecular meshwork
conventional or major pathway

Schlemm's canal

Uveoscleral
outflow
pathway

Ciliary epithelium
(aqueous production)

Figure 10.1 Diagram of the drainage angle, showing routes taken by aqueous from production to absorption.

Two theories have been advanced for the mechanism by which an elevated intraocular pressure damages nerve fibres:

1 Raised intraocular pressure causes mechanical damage to the optic nerve axons.
2 Raised intraocular pressure causes ischaemia of the nerve axons by reducing blood flow at the optic nerve head.

The pathophysiology of glaucoma is probably multifactorial, and both mechanisms are important.

Classification

The mechanism by which aqueous drainage is reduced provides a means of classifying the glaucomas. Classification of the primary glaucomas (Fig. 10.2) is based on whether or not the iris is:

- clear of the trabecular meshwork (*open angle*);
- covering the meshwork (*closed angle*).

Pathogenesis

Primary open angle glaucoma

A special contact lens (gonioscopy lens) applied to the cornea allows a view of the iridocorneal angle with the slit lamp. In open angle glaucoma the structure of the trabecular meshwork appears normal but *offers an increased resistance to the outflow* of aqueous, which results in an elevated ocular pressure. The causes of outflow obstruction include:

- thickening of the trabecular lamellae, which reduces pore size;
- reduction in the number of lining trabecular cells;
- increased extracellular material in the trabecular meshwork spaces.

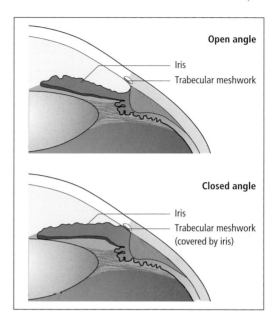

Figure 10.2 Diagram showing the difference between open and closed angle glaucoma. Outflow resistance is increased in each case. In open angle glaucoma the obstruction is due to structural changes in the trabecular meshwork. In closed angle glaucoma the peripheral iris blocks the meshwork.

Classification of the glaucomas

1 Primary glaucoma
- Chronic open angle
- Acute and chronic closed angle

2 Congenital glaucoma
- Primary
- Rubella
- Secondary to other inherited ocular disorders (e.g. aniridia – absence of the iris)

3 Secondary glaucoma (causes)
- Trauma
- Ocular surgery
- Associated with other ocular disease (e.g. uveitis)
- Raised episcleral venous pressure
- Steroid induced

A form of glaucoma also exists in which glaucomatous field loss and cupping of the optic disc occurs even though the intraocular pressure is not raised (*normal tension* or *low tension glaucoma*). It is thought that the optic nerve head in these patients is unusually susceptible to the intraocular pressure and/or has an intrinsically reduced blood flow (Fig. 10.3).

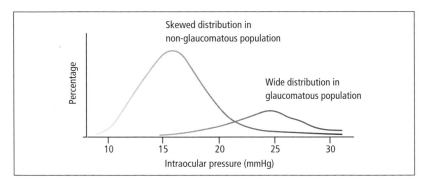

Figure 10.3 The distribution of intraocular pressure in a normal and glaucomatous population.

Conversely, intraocular pressure may be raised without evidence of visual damage or pathological optic disc cupping (*ocular hypertension*). These subjects may represent the extreme end of the normal range of intraocular pressure; however, a small proportion (about 1% per year) will subsequently develop glaucoma.

Closed angle glaucoma

The condition occurs in small eyes (i.e. often hypermetropic) with shallow anterior chambers. In the normal eye the point of contact between the pupil margin and the lens offers a resistance to aqueous flow from the posterior into the anterior chamber (relative pupil block). In angle closure glaucoma, sometimes in response to pupil dilation, when the peripheral iris may be bunched, this resistance is increased and the increased pressure gradient bows the iris forward and closes the drainage angle. Aqueous can no longer drain through the trabecular meshwork and ocular pressure rises, usually abruptly. This peripheral iris contact ultimately leads to adhesions, called *peripheral anterior synechiae* (PAS).

The severely reduced or stagnant circulation of aqueous deprives the whole cornea of nutrition and the posterior cornea of oxygen, and so gives rise to a massive degree of corneal oedema, which is amplified by the raised intraocular pressure. This results in a profound fall in vision.

However, a full-blown attack of angle closure glaucoma may be preceded by subacute episodes of angle closure, associated with transient rises of pressure, headache and oedema confined to the epithelium. In this situation, the regular separation of basal epithelial cells by oedema fluid, acting as a diffraction grating, is the basis of a key symptom of such prodromal attacks, the experience of *coloured haloes around bright lights.*

Secondary glaucoma

Intraocular pressure usually rises in secondary glaucoma due to blockage of the trabecular meshwork. The trabecular meshwork may be blocked by:

- Blood (*hyphaema*), following blunt trauma.
- Inflammatory cells (*uveitis*).
- Pigment from the iris (*pigment dispersion syndrome*).
- Deposition of material produced by the epithelium of the lens, iris and ciliary body in the trabecular meshwork (*pseudoexfoliative glaucoma*).
- Drugs increasing the resistance of the meshwork (*steroid-induced glaucoma*).

Secondary glaucoma may also result from blunt trauma to the eye damaging the drainage angle (*angle recession*).

Angle closure may also account for some cases of secondary glaucoma:

- Abnormal iris blood vessels may obstruct the angle and cause the iris to adhere to the peripheral cornea, closing the angle (*rubeosis iridis*). This may accompany proliferative diabetic retinopathy or central retinal vein occlusion due to the forward diffusion of vasoproliferative factors from the ischaemic retina (Fig. 10.4 and Chapter 12).
- A large choroidal melanoma may push the iris forward, approximating it to the peripheral cornea and causing an acute attack of angle closure glaucoma.
- A cataract may swell, pushing the iris forward and closing the drainage angle.
- Uveitis may cause the iris to adhere to the trabecular meshwork.

Raised episcleral venous pressure is an unusual cause of glaucoma but may be seen in *caroticocavernous sinus fistula*, where a connection between the carotid artery or its meningeal branches and the cavernous sinus causes a marked elevation in orbital venous pressure. It is also thought to be the cause of the raised intraocular pressure in patients with the *Sturge–Weber syndrome*.

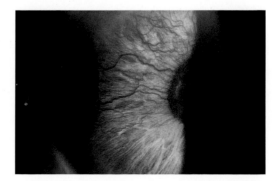

Figure 10.4 The appearance of the rubeotic iris. Note the irregular pattern of the new blood vessels on the surface.

Congenital glaucoma

The cause of congenital glaucoma remains uncertain. The iridocorneal angle may be developmentally abnormal, and covered with a membrane which increases the outflow resistance.

Chronic open angle glaucoma

Epidemiology

Chronic open angle glaucoma affects 1 in 200 of the population over the age of 40, affecting males and females equally. The prevalence increases with age to nearly 10% in the over-80 population. There may be a family history, although the exact mode of inheritance is not clear.

Genetics

First-degree relatives of patients with chronic open angle glaucoma have up to a 16% chance of developing the disease themselves. Inheritance of the condition is complex. Progress has been made with a form of the disease that presents in younger patients, juvenile open angle glaucoma (presenting at between 3 and 35 years of age). The gene (GLCIA) has been localized to the long arm of chromosome 1. There are no visible anomalies of the anterior segment, which distinguishes it from congenital glaucoma. Other gene candidates are being sought.

History

The symptoms of glaucoma depend on the rate at which intraocular pressure rises. Chronic open angle glaucoma is associated with a slow rise in pressure and is symptomless until the patient becomes aware of a visual deficit. Many patients are diagnosed when the signs of glaucoma are detected by an optometrist.

Examination

Assessment of a glaucoma suspect requires a full slit-lamp examination (Fig. 10.5):
• To measure ocular pressure with a tonometer. The normal pressure is 15.5 mmHg. The limits are defined as 2 standard deviations above and below the mean (11–21 mmHg). In chronic open angle glaucoma the pressure is typically in the 22–40 mmHg range. In angle closure glaucoma it rises above 60 mmHg.
• To measure the thickness of the cornea with a pachymeter, to adjust the value of intraocular pressure (Chapter 2).

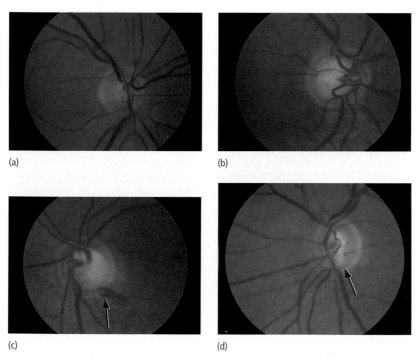

Figure 10.5 Comparison of (a) a normal optic disc, (b) a glaucomatous optic disc. (c) A disc haemorrhage (arrowed) is a feature of patients with normal tension glaucoma. (d) A glaucomatous notch (arrowed) in the disc.

- To examine the iridocorneal angle with the gonioscopy lens, to confirm that an open angle is present.
- To exclude other ocular disease that may be a secondary cause for the glaucoma.
- To examine the optic disc and determine whether it is pathologically cupped. Cupping is a normal feature of the optic disc (Fig. 10.5a). The disc is assessed by estimating the vertical ratio of the cup to the disc as a whole (the cup-to-disc ratio). In the normal eye the cup/disc ratio is usually no greater than 0.4. There is, however, a considerable range (0–0.8), and the size of the cup is related to the size of the disc. It is greater in bigger discs and less in smaller discs. In chronic glaucoma, axons entering the optic nerve head die. The central cup expands and the rim of nerve fibres (*neuroretinal rim*) becomes thinner. The nerve head becomes atrophic. The cup-to-disc ratio in the vertical becomes greater than 0.4 and the cup deepens. If the cup is deep but the cup-to-disc ratio is lower than 0.4, then chronic glaucoma is unlikely unless the disc is very small. Notching of the rim, implying focal

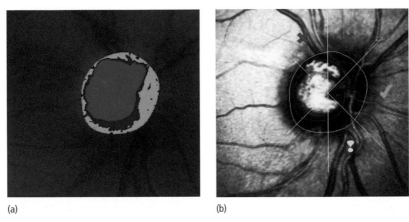

(a)   (b)

Figure 10.6 A scanning laser ophthalmoscope (Heidelberg) picture of the optic nerve head. The thin green circle in (b) outlines the optic nerve head, allowing the machine to calculate the area of the cup (red in (a)) and neuroretinal rim in different sectors of the disc.

axon loss, may also be a sign of glaucomatous damage. Defects in the nerve fibre layer of the retina may also be apparent and determines the area of field loss.

Much research is being directed towards accurate methods for analysing and recording the appearance of the disc. One involves scanning the disc with a confocal ophthalmoscope to produce an image of the disc. The neuroretinal rim area can be calculated from the image (Fig. 10.6). Other techniques record the thickness of the nerve fibre layer around the optic disc. These new technologies may help to detect changes over time, indicating whether progressive damage to the optic nerve is still occurring despite treatment.

Field testing (perimetry, see Chapter 2) is used to establish the presence of islands of field loss (*scotomata*) and to follow patients to determine whether visual damage is progressive (Fig. 10.7). A proportion of nerve fibres may, however, be damaged before field loss becomes apparent. This has stimulated the search for more sensitive means of assessing visual function with different forms of perimetry (a blue target on a yellow background instead of a white target on a white background), and testing sensitivity to motion in the peripheral visual field.

Symptoms and signs of chronic open angle glaucoma

- symptomless
- raised intraocular pressure
- visual field defect
- cupped optic disc

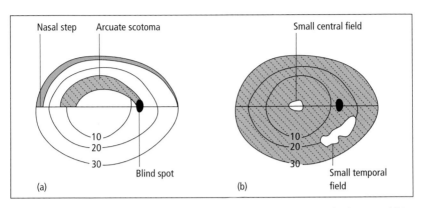

Figure 10.7 The characteristic pattern of visual field loss in chronic open angle glaucoma. (a) An upper arcuate scotoma, reflecting damage to a cohort of nerve fibres entering the lower pole of the disc (remember – the optics of the eye determine that damage to the lower retina creates an upper field defect). (b) The field loss has progressed: a small central island is left (tunnel vision), and sometimes this may be associated with sparing of an island of vision in the temporal field.

Treatment

Treatment is aimed at reducing intraocular pressure. The level to which the pressure must be lowered varies from patient to patient, and is that which minimizes further glaucomatous visual loss. This requires careful monitoring in the outpatient clinic. Three modalities of treatment are available:

1 medical treatment;
-2 laser treatment;
3 surgical treatment.

Medical treatment

Topical drugs commonly used in the treatment of glaucoma are listed in Table 10.1. In chronic open angle glaucoma the prostaglandin analogues are becoming the first-line treatment. They act by increasing the passage of aqueous through the uveoscleral pathway. Topical adrenergic beta-blockers may further reduce the pressure by suppressing aqueous secretion. Non-selective beta-blockers carry the risk of precipitating asthma through their beta-2 blocking action, following systemic absorption, or they may exacerbate an existing heart block through their beta-1 action. Beta-1 selective beta-blockers may have fewer systemic side effects, but must still be used with caution in those with respiratory disease, particularly asthma, which may be exacerbated even by the small residual beta-2 activity. If intraocular pressure remains elevated the choice lies between:

Table 10.1 Examples and mode of action of drugs used in the treatment of glaucoma. Side effects occur with variable frequency. Systemic effects are due to systemic absorption of the drug.

Drug	Action	Side effects
Topical agents		
Beta-blockers (timolol, carteolol, levobunolol, metipranolol, betaxolol-selective)	Decrease secretion	Exacerbate asthma and chronic airway disease Hypotension, bradycardia heart block
Parasympathomimetic (pilocarpine)	Increase outflow	Visual blurring in the young Darkening of the visual world due to pupillary constriction Initially, headache due to ciliary spasm
Sympathomimetic (adrenaline, dipivefrine)	Increase outflow Decrease secretion	Redness of the eye Headache palpitations
Alpha-2 agonists (apraclonidine, brimonidine)	Increase outflow through the uveoscleral pathway Decrease secretion	Redness of the eye Fatigue, drowsiness
Carbonic anhydrase inhibitors (dorzolamide, brinzolamide)	Decrease secretion	Stinging Unpleasant taste Headache
Prostaglandin analogues (latanoprost, travaprost, bimatoprost, unoprostone)	Increase outflow through the uveoscleral pathway	Increased pigmentation of the iris and periocular skin Lengthening and darkening of the lashes, conjunctival hyperaemia Rarely, macular oedema, uveitis
Systemic agents		
Carbonic anhydrase inhibitors (acetazolamide)	Decrease secretion	Tingling in limbs Depression, sleepiness Renal stones Stevens–Johnson syndrome

- adding additional medical treatment;
- laser treatment;
- surgical drainage procedures.

Laser trabeculoplasty

This involves placing a series of laser burns (50 μm wide) in the trabecular mesh-work, to improve aqueous outflow. Whilst effective initially, the intraocular pressure may slowly increase. In the UK there is an increasing tendency to proceed to early drainage surgery.

Surgical treatment

Drainage surgery (*trabeculectomy*) relies on the creation of a fistula between the anterior chamber and the subconjunctival space (Fig. 10.8). The operation usually achieves a substantial reduction in intraocular pressure. It is performed increasingly early in the treatment of glaucoma.

Complications of surgery include·

- shallowing of the anterior chamber in the immediate postoperative period risking damage to the lens and cornea;
- intraocular infection;
- possibly accelerated cataract development;
- failure to reduce intraocular pressure adequately.
- an excessively low pressure (hypotony) which may cause macular oedema.

Evidence suggests that some topical medications, particularly those containing sympathomimetic agents or preservatives, may decrease the success of surgery by causing increased postoperative subconjunctival scarring, resulting in a non-functional drainage channel. In patients particularly prone to scarring, anti-metabolite drugs (5-fluorouracil and mitomycin) may be used at the time of surgery to prevent fibrosis.

Recent research has examined the benefit of modifying the trabeculectomy operation by removing the sclera under the scleral flap but not making a fistula into the anterior chamber (*deep sclerostomy*, *viscocanalostomy*). The long-term benefit of the procedure is being assessed.

Normal tension glaucoma

Normal tension glaucoma, considered to lie at one end of the spectrum of chronic open angle glaucoma, can be particularly difficult to treat. Some patients appear to have non-progressive visual field defects and require no treatment. In those with progressive field loss, lowering intraocular pressure may be beneficial.

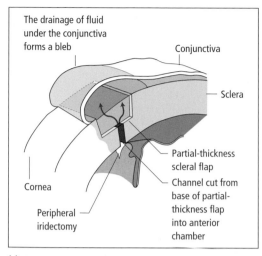

The drainage of fluid under the conjunctiva forms a bleb

Conjunctiva

Sclera

Partial-thickness scleral flap

Channel cut from base of partial-thickness flap into anterior chamber

Cornea

Peripheral iridectomy

(a)

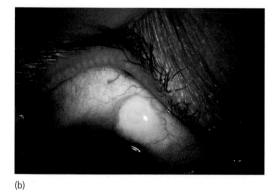

(b)

Figure 10.8 (a) Diagram showing a section through a trabeculectomy. An incision is made in the conjunctiva, which is dissected and reflected to expose bare sclera. A partial-thickness scleral flap is then fashioned. Just anterior to the scleral spur a small opening (termed a *sclerostomy*) is made into the anterior chamber to create a low-resistance channel for aqueous. The iris is excised in the region of the sclerostomy (*iridectomy*) to prevent it moving forward and blocking the opening. The partial-thickness flap is loosely sutured back into place. The conjunctiva is tightly sutured. Aqueous can now leak through the sclerostomy, around and through the scleral flap and underneath the conjunctiva, where it forms a bleb. (b) The appearance of a trabeculectomy bleb.

Each form of treatment has its complications, and therapy must be aimed at minimizing these whilst maximizing effectiveness.

Primary angle closure glaucoma

Epidemiology

Primary angle closure glaucoma affects 1 in 1000 subjects over 40 years old, with females more commonly affected than males. Patients with angle closure glaucoma are likely to be long-sighted, because the long-sighted eye is small and the structures of the anterior chamber are more crowded.

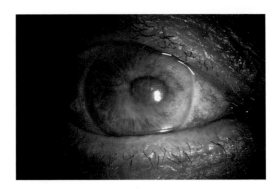

Figure 10.9 The appearance of the eye in angle closure glaucoma. Note the cloudy cornea and dilated pupil.

History

In acute angle closure glaucoma, there is an abrupt increase in pressure and the eye becomes photophobic and very painful due to ischaemic tissue damage. There is watering of the eye and loss of vision. The patient may be systemically unwell with nausea and abdominal pain, symptoms which may take them to a general casualty department.

Intermittent primary angle closure glaucoma occurs when an acute attack spontaneously resolves. The patient may complain of pain, blurring of vision and seeing haloes around lights.

Examination

On examination visual acuity is reduced, the eye red, the cornea cloudy and the pupil oval, fixed and dilated (Fig. 10.9).

Treatment

The acute and dramatic rise in pressure seen in angle closure glaucoma must be urgently countered to prevent permanent damage to the vision. Acetazolamide is administered intravenously and subsequently orally, together with topical pilocarpine and beta-blockers. Pilocarpine constricts the pupil and draws the peripheral iris out of the angle; the acetazolamide and beta-blocker reduce aqueous secretion and the pressure gradient across the iris. These measures often break the attack and lower intraocular pressure. Subsequent management requires that a small hole (*iridotomy* or *iridectomy*) be made in the peripheral iris to prevent subsequent attacks. This provides an alternative pathway for fluid to flow from the posterior to the anterior chamber, thus reducing the pressure gradient across the iris. This can be done with a YAG laser or surgically.

If the pressure has been raised for some days the iris becomes adherent to the peripheral cornea (*peripheral anterior synechiae* or *PAS*). The iridocorneal angle is damaged, and additional medical or surgical measures may be required to lower the ocular pressure. In some patients with cataract, lens extraction with implantation of an intraocular lens may help open the iridocorneal angle.

Secondary glaucoma

Secondary glaucomas are much rarer than the primary glaucomas. The symptoms and signs depend on the rate at which intraocular pressure rises; most are again symptomless. Treatment broadly follows the lines of the primary disease. In secondary glaucoma it is important to treat any underlying cause, e.g. uveitis, which may be responsible for the glaucoma.

In particularly difficult cases it may be necessary to selectively ablate the ciliary processes in order to reduce aqueous production. This is done by application of a laser or cryoprobe to the sclera overlying the processes. Endoscopic techniques are also under development.

Congenital glaucoma

This covers a diverse range of disease. It may present at birth or within the first year. Symptoms and signs include:
- excessive tearing;
- an increased corneal diameter (*buphthalmos*);
- a cloudy cornea due to epithelial oedema;
- splits in Descemet's membrane.

Congenital glaucoma is usually treated surgically. An incision is made into the trabecular meshwork (*goniotomy*) to increase aqueous drainage, or a direct passage between Schlemm's canal and the anterior chamber is created (*trabeculotomy*).

Prognosis of the glaucomas

The goal of treatment in glaucoma is to stop or reduce the rate of visual damage. It may be that control of intraocular pressure alone is not the only factor that needs to be addressed in the management of glaucoma. The possible role of optic nerve ischaemia has been discussed, and there is interest in developing neuro protective drugs. Reducing intraocular pressure is thus currently the mainstay of treatment. Some patients will continue to develop visual loss despite a large decrease in intraocular pressure. Nonetheless vigorous lowering of intraocular pressure, even when it does not prevent continued visual loss, appears to significantly reduce the rate of progression. If the diagnosis is made late, when there is already

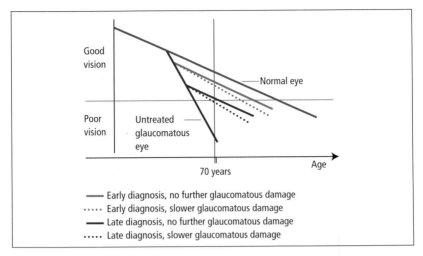

Figure 10.10 All eyes suffer a gradual loss of neurones with aging but death normally precedes a visually significant decline. In glaucoma this loss is speeded up and visually significant loss may occur during life (red line). Early diagnosis of the condition with lowering of intraocular pressure results in future age-related neuronal loss only (green line parallel to the normal eye). Even if there is some continued glaucomatous damage the rate is slowed and the patient is unlikely to suffer visual loss during their lifetime (interrupted green line). If the diagnosis is made late (purple lines), arresting the glaucoma completely may still result in visual loss during the patient's lifetime. This emphasizes the need for early diagnosis.

significant visual damage, the eye is more likely to become blind despite treatment (Fig. 10.10).

If intraocular pressure remains controlled following acute treatment of angle closure glaucoma, progressive visual damage is unlikely. The same applies to the secondary glaucomas, if treatment of the underlying cause results in a reduction of intraocular pressure into the normal range.

Key points

- Glaucoma is an optic neuropathy caused by an elevation of intraocular pressure.
- Primary glaucoma is classified according to whether the trabecular meshwork is obstructed by the peripheral iris (angle closure) or not (open angle glaucoma).
- Treatment of glaucoma relies on lowering ocular pressure to reduce or prevent further visual damage.
- Ocular pressure can be reduced with topical and systemic medications, laser treatment and surgery.
- Beware patients who are acutely debilitated with a red eye; they may have acute angle closure glaucoma.

Multiple choice questions

1. Which of the following statements are true?

a Aqueous is produced by the ciliary processes. The fluid circulates through the pupil and is drained by the trabecular meshwork.

b The uveoscleral pathway accounts for most of the drainage of aqueous.

c The major classification of glaucoma depends on the anatomy of the iridocorneal angle.

d One mechanism of angle closure glaucoma is an increased resistance to aqueous flow through the pupil. This causes the iris to bow forwards and block the drainage angle.

e Glaucoma is always associated with a raised pressure.

2. A patient is found by his optician to have an arcuate visual field defect, an enlarged optic cup and raised intraocular pressure.

a The most likely diagnosis is acute glaucoma.

b The most likely diagnosis is chronic open angle glaucoma.

c Treatment is with intravenous acetazolamide.

d Treatment is confined to topical therapy.

e The corneal diameter will be increased.

3. A patient presents to casualty with a painful red eye and a cloudy cornea. The casualty officer suspects he has acute glaucoma.

a He should arrange for him to be seen in the eye clinic in a week.

b The diagnosis would be further confirmed by finding a dilated pupil.

c Treatment is initially with intravenous acetazolamide and pilocarpine eye drops.

d A laser iridotomy should be performed.

e The condition may be caused by a block to the flow of aqueous through the pupil.

4. Symptoms of congenital glaucoma include

a A watering eye.

b Increased corneal diameter.

c A red eye.

d Splits in Descemet's membrane.

e Cloudiness of the cornea.

5. Glaucoma surgery (trabeculectomy)

a May be complicated by intraocular infection.

b Is associated with accelerated cataract development.

c Retinal detachment is a common complication of the surgery.

d Reverses damage to the optic nerve caused by glaucoma.

e Success of surgery may be improved by using antimetabolites topically.

6. Match the side effects of treatment with the drug class

a Exacerbation of asthma.

b Visual blurring in patients with cataract.

c Redness of the eye, increased pigmentation of the periocular skin, darkening of the iris, lengthening of the eyelashes.

d Tingling in the fingers and around the mouth.

  i Beta-blockers.

  ii Prostaglandin analogues.

  iii Parasympathomimetic agents.

  iv Systemic carbonic anhydrase inhibitors.

Answers

1. Which of the following statements are true?

a True.

b False. The uveoscleral pathway accounts for only a small proportion of flow. The conventional pathway across the trabecular meshwork accounts for most of the outflow.

c True. Glaucoma is essentially classified into open and closed angle glaucoma.

d True.

e False. Some patients develop the typical signs of glaucoma (glaucomatous field loss and disc cupping) but have an intraocular pressure within the normal range.

2. A patient is found by his optician to have an arcuate visual field defect, an enlarged optic cup and raised intraocular pressure.

a False. This is an acute painful condition.

b True.

c False. Intravenous acetazolamide is used to suppress aqueous secretion quickly, in acute glaucoma.

d False. Although this is the commonest treatment, laser and surgical treatments are also possible.

e False. This is only seen in congenital glaucoma.

3. A patient presents to casualty with a painful red eye and a cloudy cornea. The casualty officer suspects he has acute glaucoma.

a False. The patient must be referred immediately for treatment.

b True.

c True.

d True. This is the definitive treatment.

e True.

4. Symptoms of congenital glaucoma include

a True.

b True.

c False.

d True.

e True.

5. Glaucoma surgery (trabeculectomy)

a True. This is a potential complication of any intraocular surgery.

b True.

c False.

d False. No treatment is known to reverse the damage of glaucoma, but the rate of progression can be reduced with treatment.

e True. A topical antimetabolite, applied to the sclera at the time of surgery, reduces scarring and allows a functioning drainage bleb to form.

6. Match the side effects of treatment with the drug class

a Beta-blockers (i).

b Parasympathomimetic agents (iii).

c Prostaglandin analogues (ii).

d Systemic carbonic anhydrase inhibitors (iv).

Chapter 11

Retina and choroid

Learning objectives

To understand:
- The symptoms of retinal disease.
- The cause and treatment of acquired and inherited retinal disease.
- The symptoms, signs and complications of posterior vitreous detachment.
- The symptoms, signs, complications and treatment of retinal detachment.
- The symptoms, signs and treatment of retinal and choroidal tumours.

Introduction

The retina is subject to an enormous range of disease, both inherited and acquired. Some are common, with significant socioeconomic importance (e.g. age-related macular degeneration), while others are much rarer (for example some of the macular dystrophies). The impact on the individual may be profound in either case. Diseases of the macula, particularly if bilateral, result in a profound reduction in visual acuity. Despite the variety of diseases, the symptoms are relatively stereotyped. These will be described first. In this chapter both hereditary and acquired disease of the vitreous, neuroretina, retinal pigment epithelium and choroid will be described. In the chapter which follows the effects of disorders of the retinal circulation will be explored.

Symptoms of retinal disease

Macular dysfunction

The central part of the macula (*the fovea*) is responsible for fine resolution. Disorders of this relatively small part of the retina cause significant visual impairment. The patient may complain of:

• Blurred central vision.

• Distorted vision (*metamorphopsia*) caused by a disturbance in the arrangement of the photoreceptors such as that which occurs in macular oedema. A reduction (*micropsia*) or enlargement (*macropsia*) of object size may also occur if the photoreceptors become stretched apart or compressed together.

• The patient may notice areas of loss of the central visual field (*scotomata*) if part of the photoreceptor layer becomes covered, e.g. by blood, or if the photoreceptors are destroyed.

Peripheral retinal dysfunction

The patient complains of:

• Loss of visual field (usually detected clinically when a significant amount of the peripheral retina is damaged). Small areas of damage, e.g. small haemorrhages, do not produce clinically detectable defects. The field loss may be absolute, for example in a branch retinal artery occlusion, or relative (i.e. brighter or larger objects are visible) as in a retinal detachment.

• Some diseases affecting the retina may predominantly affect one type of photoreceptor; in retinitis pigmentosa the rods are principally affected so that night vision is reduced (night blindness).

Acquired macular disease

Acquired disease at the macula may destroy part or all of the thickness of the retina (e.g. age-related macular degeneration or a macular hole). In a number of conditions this damage is dramatically magnified by the growth of new vessels from the choroid through Bruch's membrane and the retinal pigment epithelium, causing haemorrhage or exudation of fluid into the sub-retinal space and subsequent scarring of the retina. The neuro retina ceases to function if it is detached from the retinal pigment epithelium, so these changes cause marked disruption of macular function even before direct retinal damage occurs.

Fluid may also accumulate within the layers of the retina at the macula (*cystoid macular oedema*) if the normal tight junctions of the retinal capillaries that form the inner blood–retina barrier break down. This may occur following intraocular surgery, such as cataract surgery. The retina and sub-retinal layers may also become separated by diffusion of fluid from the choriocapillaris through an abnormal region of the retinal pigment epithelium. This represents a breakdown of the outer blood–retinal barrier between the choroid and the retina, and is termed central serous retinopathy. It may occur unilaterally, as a potentially reversible disorder in young men.

Age-related macular degeneration

Age-related macular degeneration (AMD) is the commonest cause of irreversible visual loss in the developed world (Fig. 11.1).

Pathogenesis

The retinal pigment epithelium (RPE) removes and processes the used discs of the photoreceptor outer segments. Over time, undigested lipid products, such as the

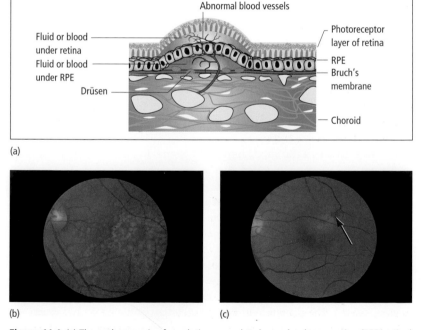

Figure 11.1 (a) The pathogenesis of exudative age-related macular degeneration (RPE, retinal pigment epithelium). Pictures of: (b) dry AMD: note the discrete scattered yellowish sub-retinal drüsen; (c) wet AMD: note the small haemorrhage associated with the sub-retinal membrane.

age pigment lipofuscin, accumulate in the RPE and the excess material is transferred to Bruch's membrane, impairing its diffusional properties. Deposits form in Bruch's membrane which can be seen with the ophthalmoscope as discrete, subretinal yellow lesions called drüsen. Collections of these drüsen in the macula give rise to the condition termed *age-related maculopathy* or ARM. The neighbouring RPE and photoreceptors may also show degenerative changes, producing the dry or non-exudative form of age-related macular degeneration (AMD). In the less common exudative or 'wet' form, new vessels from the choroid, stimulated by angiogenic factors such as vascular endothelial growth factor (VEGF), grow through Bruch's membrane and the RPE into the sub-retinal space, where they form a *sub-retinal neovascular membrane*. Subsequent haemorrhage into the sub-retinal space or even through the retina into the vitreous is associated with profound visual loss.

Symptoms

The symptoms are those of macular dysfunction outlined above.

Signs

The usual foveal reflex is absent. Yellow, well-circumscribed drüsen may be seen, and there may be areas of hypo- and hyperpigmentation. In exudative AMD sub-retinal, or more occasionally pre-retinal, haemorrhages may be seen. The experienced observer may detect elevation of the retina stereoscopically.

Investigation

Diagnosis is based on the appearance of the retina. In patients with a suspected exudative AMD and with vision that is not severely affected, a fluorescein angiogram is performed to delineate the position of the sub-retinal neovascular membrane. The position of the membrane determines whether or not the patient may benefit from laser treatment.

Treatment

There is no treatment for non-exudative AMD. Vision is maximized with low-vision aids including magnifiers and telescopes and closed-circuit television devices (CCTV). The patient must be reassured that although central vision has been lost, the disease will not spread to affect the peripheral vision. Therefore navigational vision is retained. This is a vital message, since many patients fear that they will become totally blind.

In a small proportion of patients with exudative AMD, where the fluorescein angiogram reveals a sub-retinal vascular membrane eccentric to the fovea, it is possible to obliterate it with argon-laser treatment. Subfoveal vascular membranes cannot be treated by conventional argon lasers since the energy is sufficient to damage the overlying photoreceptors responsible for central visual acuity. However they can be safely obliterated by photodynamic therapy (PDT), which involves the intravenous injection of a porphyrin-like dye (indocyanine green) that is activated by a non-thermal laser beam as it traverses the blood vessels of the membrane. The activated molecules destroy the vessels but spare the nearby photoreceptors. Unfortunately even with laser treatment the condition can recur, in which case treatment must be repeated.

Recent clinical trials have shown that drugs inhibiting the action of angiogenic factors such as VEGF and steroids may be effective in the treatment of exudative AMD by retarding angiogenesis and causing regression of existing vessels. These anti-VEGF agents are currently given by repeated injections into the vitreous. They reduce visual loss and restore the normal anatomical appearance of the macula.

Other degenerative conditions associated with the formation of sub-retinal neovascular membranes

- Degenerative changes and sub-retinal neovascular membranes may also occur at the maculae of very myopic patients and can cause loss of central vision, particularly in young adulthood.
- Sub-retinal neovascular membranes may also grow through elongated cracks in Bruch's membrane called *angioid streaks* (Fig. 11.2). These are seen classically in the rare recessive disorder pseudoxanthoma elasticum, and uncommonly in systemic diseases such as Paget's disease and sickle cell disease. Again there may be a

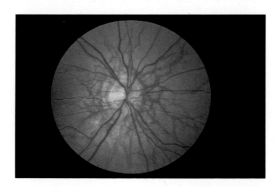

Figure 11.2 The clinical appearance of angioid streaks in pseudoxanthoma elasticum.

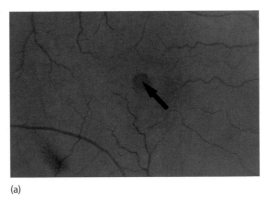

(a)

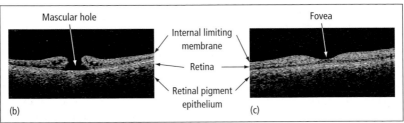

Figure 11.3 (a) The appearance of a macular hole. (b) An optical coherence tomogram (OCT) scan of the retina showing a macular hole, compared to (c) a normal scan.

profound reduction in central vision. Vision is also reduced if the crack itself passes through the fovea.

Macular holes and membranes

A well-circumscribed hole may form at the centre of the macular region and destroy the fovea, resulting in a major loss of acuity (Fig. 11.3). It results from vitreous traction on the thin macular retina. The early stages of hole formation may be associated with visual distortion and mild blurring of vision.

Unlike peripheral retinal holes, macular holes are not usually associated with retinal detachment. Most are idiopathic in origin, but they may be associated with blunt trauma. Much interest is being shown in the treatment of macular holes with vitreous surgery to relieve the traction on the retina. No other treatment is available.

A pre-retinal glial membrane may form over the macular region, whose contraction causes puckering of the retina and again results in blurring and distortion of vision. These symptoms may be improved by removing the membrane with microsurgical vitrectomy techniques.

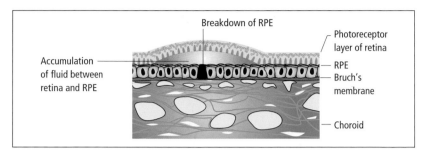

Figure 11.4 The pattern of fluid accumulation in central serous retinopathy.

Central serous retinopathy

This localized accumulation of fluid between the neuro retina and the RPE separates the two layers and causes distortion of the photoreceptor layer. It results from a localized breakdown in the normal structure of the RPE. It is usually unilateral and typically affects young or middle-aged males. Patients complain of distortion and blurred vision. Examination reveals a dome-shaped elevation of the retina (Fig. 11.4).

Treatment is not usually required, as the condition is self-limiting. Occasionally, in intractable cases or those where the vision is severely affected, the argon laser can be used to seal the point of leakage identified with a fluorescein angiogram.

Macular oedema

This accumulation of fluid within the retina itself is a further cause of distorted and blurred vision (Fig. 11.5). Ophthalmoscopy reveals a loss of the normal foveal reflex and with experience a rather cystic appearance to the fovea. If the diagnosis is in doubt a confirmatory OCT scan (Fig. 11.5) or a fluorescein angiogram can be performed. The fluorescein leaks out into the oedematous retina (see Chapter 2).

Macular oedema may be associated with numerous and diverse eye disorders, including:
- intraocular surgery;
- uveitis;
- retinal vascular disease (e.g. diabetic retinopathy);
- retinitis pigmentosa.

Treatment can be difficult and is dependent on the associated eye disease. Steroids in high doses are helpful in macular oedema caused by uveitis; acetazolamide may be helpful in treating patients with retinitis pigmentosa or following intraocular surgery.

Prolonged macular oedema can cause the formation of a lamellar macular hole.

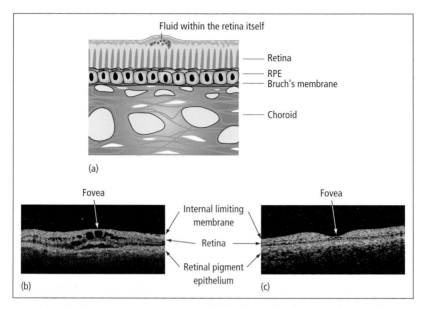

Figure 11.5 (a) The pattern of fluid accumulation in macular oedema (schematic). (b) An optical coherence tomogram (OCT) scan showing cysts of fluid in the retina of a patient with macular oedema, compared to (c) a normal scan.

Toxic maculopathies

The accumulation of some drugs in the RPE can cause macular damage. These include the antimalarials chloroquine and hydroxychloroquine, used quite widely in the treatment of rheumatoid arthritis and other connective-tissue disorders, which may cause a toxic maculopathy. Chloroquine is the more toxic. Patients on chloroquine require regular visual assessment for maculopathy (Fig. 11.6). The maculopathy is initially only detected by accurate assessment of macular function. At this early stage, discontinuation of the drug reverses the maculopathy. Later, a pigmentary target lesion is seen ophthalmoscopically, associated with metamorphopsia and an appreciable and irreversible loss of central vision. Ocular toxicity is unlikely with a dose of less than 4 mg (chloroquine phosphate) per kg lean body weight per day or a total cumulative dose of less than 300 g. Screening of patients on hydroxychloroquine, although still advised, is questioned by some.

Phenothiazines (thioridazine particularly) used in high doses for prolonged periods (to treat psychoses) may cause retinal damage.

Tamoxifen, in high doses, may cause a maculopathy.

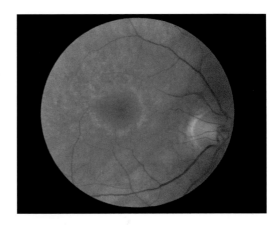

Figure 11.6 Bull's-eye appearance in chloroquine maculopathy.

Vitreous floaters and posterior vitreous detachment

The vitreous undergoes degenerative changes in patients in their 50s and 60s (earlier in myopes), with the formation of fragments of condensed vitreous which cast shadows on the retina, giving rise to the common symptom of vitreous 'floaters'. These take the form of spots or cobwebs which obscure vision only slightly and move when the eyes move, reflecting the fluid nature of the vitreous. Symptoms are most marked on bright days, when the small pupil throws a sharper image on the retina.

Sometimes, in older patients or myopes, the vitreous gel collapses and detaches from points of retinal attachment, a condition termed a *posterior vitreous detachment* (Fig. 11.7). This gives rise to acute symptoms of:

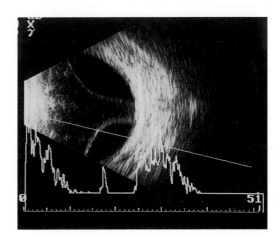

Figure 11.7 Ultrasound picture showing a posterior vitreous detachment. Note that the vitreous is still attached at the optic disc.

- *Photopsia* (flashing lights) – due to traction on the retina by the detaching vitreous.
- A shower of floaters – representing condensations within the collapsed vitreous, or sometimes a vitreous haemorrhage caused when the detaching vitreous ruptures a small blood vessel during the formation of a retinal tear or hole.

For this reason presentation with symptoms of an acute vitreous detachment is an indication for full assessment of the vitreous and peripheral retina with full pupil dilation.

Retinal detachment

Pathogenesis

The potential space between the neuroretina and its pigment epithelium corresponds to the cavity of the embryonic optic vesicle. The two tissues are loosely attached in the mature eye and may become separated:

- If a tear occurs in the retina, allowing liquefied vitreous to gain entry to the sub-retinal space and causing a progressive detachment (*rhegmatogenous retinal detachment* this may be partial or total).
- If it is pulled off by contracting fibrous tissue on the retinal surface, e.g. in the proliferative retinopathy of diabetes mellitus (*traction retinal detachment*).
- When, rarely, fluid accumulates in the sub-retinal space as a result of an exudative process, which may occur with retinal tumours or during toxaemia of pregnancy (*exudative retinal detachment*).

Tears in the retina are most commonly associated with the onset of a posterior vitreous detachment. As the gel separates from the retina the traction it exerts (*vitreous traction*) becomes more localized and thus greater. Occasionally it may be sufficient to tear the retina. An underlying peripheral weakness of the retina such as *lattice degeneration* increases the probability of a tear forming when the vitreous pulls on the retina. Highly myopic people have a significantly increased risk of developing retinal detachment.

Rhegmatogenous retinal detachment

Epidemiology

About 1 in 10 000 of the normal population will suffer a rhegmatogenous retinal detachment (Fig. 11.8). The probability is increased in patients who:

- are high myopes;
- have undergone cataract surgery, particularly if this was complicated by vitreous loss;

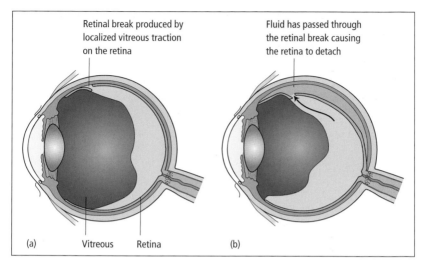

Retinal break produced by localized vitreous traction on the retina

Fluid has passed through the retinal break causing the retina to detach

(a)   Vitreous   Retina   (b)

Figure 11.8 The formation of a rhegmatogenous retinal detachment. (a) The detaching vitreous has torn the retina; the vitreous continues to pull on the retina surrounding the break (vitreous traction). (b) Fluid from the vitreous cavity passes through the break, detaching the neuro retina from the underlying retinal pigment epithelium.

- have experienced a detached retina in the fellow eye;
- have been subjected to recent severe eye trauma.

Symptoms

Retinal detachment may be preceded by symptoms of a posterior vitreous detachment, including floaters and flashing lights. With the onset of the retinal detachment itself the patient notices the progressive development of a field defect, often described as a 'shadow' or 'curtain'. Progression may be rapid when a superior detachment is present. If the macula becomes detached there is a marked fall in visual acuity.

Signs

The detached retina is visible on ophthalmoscopy as a floating, diaphonous membrane which partly obscures the choroidal vascular detail. If there is a marked accumulation of fluid in the sub-retinal space (a *bullous retinal detachment*) undulating movements of the retina will be observed as the eye moves. A tear in the retina appears reddish pink because of the underlying choroidal vessels. There may be

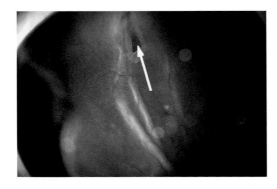

Figure 11.9 The clinical appearance of a retinal detachment. Note the retinal tear. The retina has completely detached.

associated debris in the vitreous comprising blood (*vitreous haemorrhage*) and pigment, or the lid (*operculum*) of a retinal hole may be found floating free (Fig. 11.9).

Management

There are two major surgical techniques for repairing a retinal detachment (Fig. 11.10):
1 external (*conventional approach*);
2 internal (*vitreoretinal surgery*).
The essential principle behind both techniques is to close the causative break in the retina and to increase the strength of attachment between the surrounding retina and the retinal pigment epithelium by inducing inflammation in the region, either by local freezing with a cryoprobe or with a laser. In the external approach the break is closed by indenting the sclera with an externally located strip of silicone plomb (or sponge). This relieves the vitreous traction on the retinal hole and apposes the retinal pigment epithelium with the retina. It may first be necessary to drain an extensive accumulation of sub-retinal fluid by piercing the sclera and choroid with a needle (*sclerostomy*).

In the internal approach the vitreous is removed with a special microsurgical cutter introduced into the vitreous cavity through the pars plana, and this relieves the vitreous traction on the break. Fluid can be drained through the causative retinal break itself, and laser or cryotherapy applied to the surrounding retina. A temporary internal tamponade is then obtained by injecting an inert fluorocarbon gas into the vitreous cavity which is absorbed slowly. This has the effect of closing the hole from the inside and preventing further passage of fluid through the break. The patient has to maintain a particular head posture for a few days to ensure that the bubble continuously covers the retinal break. Air travel must be avoided with the gas in place.

Retinal tears not associated with sub-retinal fluid are treated prophylactically with a laser or cryoprobe to induce inflammation and increase the adhesion

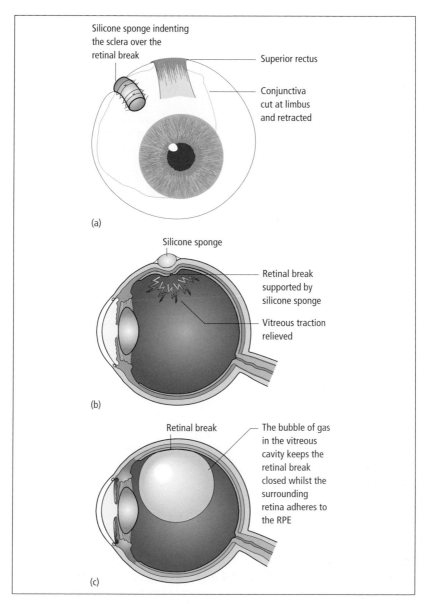

Figure 11.10 The repair of a retinal detachment. (a) External approach: a silicone sponge has been sutured to the globe to indent the sclera over the retinal break following drainage of the sub-retinal fluid and application of cryotherapy; (b) sagittal section of the eye showing the indent formed by the silicone sponge: the retina is now reattached and traction on the retinal break by the vitreous is relieved. (c) Internal approach: following removal of the vitreous gel and drainage of sub-retinal fluid an inert fluorocarbon gas has been injected into the vitreous cavity.

between the neuro retina surrounding the tear and the pigment epithelium, thus preventing a retinal detachment. It is always important to check the peripheral retina in the fellow eye, as tears or an asymptomatic retinal detachment may be seen here too.

Prognosis

If the macula is attached and the surgery successfully reattaches the peripheral retina the outlook for vision is excellent. If the macula is detached for more than 24 hours prior to surgery the previous visual acuity will probably not recover completely. Nonetheless a substantial part of the vision may be restored over several months. If the retina is not successfully attached and the surgery is complicated, then fibrotic changes may occur in the vitreous (*proliferative vitreoretinopathy, PVR*), which may cause traction on the retina and further retinal detachment. A complex vitreoretinal procedure may permit vision to be retained, but the outlook for vision is much poorer.

Traction retinal detachment

The neuro retina is pulled away from the pigment epithelium by contracting fibrous tissue which has grown on the retinal surface. This may be seen in proliferative diabetic retinopathy or may occur as a result of proliferative vitreoretinopathy. Vitreoretinal surgery is required to repair these detachments. In these cases it may be necessary to inject silicone oil into the vitreous cavity to help hold the retina flat.

Retinoschisis

The retina splits into an inner and outer leaf at the outer plexiform and inner nuclear junction. It is usually seen in the lower temporal quadrant of the retina and is often bilateral. The appearance is not dissimilar to a retinal detachment. It may, but rarely does, cause a retinal detachment when there are holes in both the inner and outer leaves.

Inherited retinal dystrophies and photoreceptor dystrophies

Retinitis pigmentosa

Retinitis pigmentosa is an inherited disorder of the photoreceptors which has several genotypic and phenotypic varieties. It may occur in isolation or in association with a number of other systemic diseases.

Pathogenesis

The disease affects both types of photoreceptors, but the rods are particularly affected. The inheritance may be:

- autosomal recessive (sporadic cases are often in this category);
- autosomal dominant;
- X-linked recessive.

Several forms of retinitis pigmentosa have been shown to be due to mutations in the gene for rhodopsin.

Epidemiology

The prevalence of this group of diseases is 1 in 4000.

Symptoms

The age of onset, progression and prognosis are dependent on the mode of inheritance. In general the dominant form is of later onset and milder degree, while recessive and X-linked recessive forms may present in infancy or childhood. Patients notice poor night vision, visual fields become increasingly constricted, and central vision may ultimately be lost.

Signs

The three signs of typical retinitis pigmentosa (Fig. 11.11) are:

1 peripheral clumps of retinal pigmentation (termed 'bone spicule' pigmentation);
2 attenuation of the retinal arterioles;
3 disc pallor.

Patients may also have cataracts at an early age and may develop macular oedema.

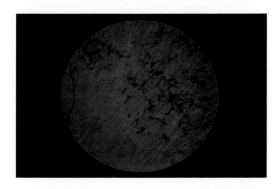

Figure 11.11 The clinical appearance of the peripheral retina in retinitis pigmentosa.

Investigation

A careful family history will help to determine the mode of inheritance. The diagnosis can usually be made clinically. Electrophysiologic tests are also useful in diagnosis, particularly in early disease, where there may be few clinical signs.

Recent work on mapping the genetic loci for the condition has opened new avenues for genetic counselling and determining disease mechanism.

The possibility of associated syndromes should be borne in mind. Usher's syndrome, for example, is a recessive disorder characterized by deafness and retinitis pigmentosa. Retinitis pigmentosa also occurs in mitochondrial disease.

Management

Unfortunately nothing can be done to prevent the progression of the disease. Associated ocular problems can be treated. Cataracts can be removed, and macular oedema may respond to treatment with acetazolamide. Low-vision aids may be helpful for a period. The possibility of genetic counselling should be discussed with the patient.

Prognosis

X-linked recessive and autosomal recessive disease produce the most severe visual symptoms. About 50% of all patients with retinitis pigmentosa will have an acuity of less than 6/60 by the time they reach 50.

Cone dystrophy

This is less common than retinitis pigmentosa. It is usually autosomal dominant, but many cases are sporadic. Patients present in the first decade of life with poor vision. Examination reveals an abnormal, banded macular appearance which has been likened to a bull's-eye target. No treatment is possible but it is important to provide appropriate help, not only to help maximize vision but also to help with educational problems. Genetic counselling should be offered.

Juvenile macular dystrophies

There are a variety of inherited conditions that affect both the retinal pigment epithelium and, secondarily, the photoreceptors. All are rare (e.g. the recessive disorder *Stargardt's dystrophy*) and the prognosis for vision is often poor. Once again the social and educational needs of the patient need to be assessed and genetic counselling offered.

Albinism

These patients have defective melanin synthesis. There are two types:
1 Ocular albinism, where the lack of pigmentation is confined to the eye. There are X-linked and recessive forms.
2 Oculocutaneous albinism, a recessive disorder where the hair is white and the skin is pale; a few of these patients can manufacture some melanin.
Clinically the iris is blue and there is marked transillumination so that the red reflex is seen through the iris because of the lack of pigmentation; this also allows the lens edge to be viewed through the iris. The fundus appears abnormal, with lack of a normal foveal reflex, extreme pallor and prominent visibility of the choroidal vessels. Vision is poor from birth and patients often have nystagmus. There is an abnormal projection of retinal axons to the lateral geniculate bodies.

Some patients will have associated systemic disease (e.g. the Hermansky–Pudlak syndrome, where there is an associated haemorrhagic diathesis).

Retinal tumours

Retinoblastoma

This is the commonest malignant tumour of the eye in childhood, with a frequency of 1 per 20 000 births. It may be inherited as an autosomal dominant condition, but most cases are sporadic. Retinoblastoma is caused either by germinal mutations, which can be passed on to the next generation, or by somatic mutations in a single retinal cell, which cannot be genetically transmitted (the majority, some 66% of cases). The retinoblastoma gene is a tumour suppressor gene whose product (pRB) plays a key role in the cell cycle as a negative regulator of cell proliferation. Mutations remove this anti-proliferative action. The disease is initiated in fetal retinal cells exhibiting a *homozygous defect* in the retinoblastoma gene. In inherited retinoblastoma one mutation is inherited and the other occurs by spontaneous somatic mutation in the retina during development. The mutation rate for the gene is thought to be 1 : 10 000 000, and 100 000 000 divisions are needed to form the adult retina – so the chance of a somatic mutation occurring in a subject with only one functioning gene is very high. For this reason, inherited retinoblastoma is frequently bilateral. The homozygous state is thus achieved by a *'double hit'* event and the condition behaves as a *pseudodominant disorder*. The chance of developing retinoblastoma (the penetrance) in a child inheriting the genetic trait is 85%. Thus, although it occurs frequently in affected families, there may be some skip generations. Sporadic retinoblastoma occurs when two spontaneous mutations occur by chance in the same primordial retinal cell. Because the chances of this occurring are low, this form of retinoblastoma is most commonly unilateral.

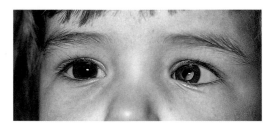

Figure 11.12 Left leucocoria.

History and symptoms

The child may present (at a mean age of 8 months if inherited and 25 months if sporadic) with:

• A white pupillary reflex (*leucocoria*) due to a pale elevated tumour at the posterior pole of the eye (Fig. 11.12). Sometimes the tumour is bilateral on presentation.

• A squint due to reduced vision.

• Occasionally, a painful red eye.

Most cases present by the age of two. Inherited retinoblastoma is often bilateral. When the condition is unilateral on presentation and there is no family history, inherited disease is less likely, but not excluded.

Signs

Dilated fundoscopy shows a whitish-pink mass protruding from the retina into the vitreous cavity.

Investigations

The diagnosis is usually a clinical one. Cerebrospinal fluid and bone marrow must be examined to check for metastatic disease.

Treatment

Removal (enucleation) of the eye is performed in advanced cases. Radiotherapy can be used in less advanced disease, as can cryotherapy and photocoagulation. Metastatic disease (either by direct spread through the optic nerve or by a haematogenous route) is treated with chemotherapy. Regular follow-up of an affected child is required. Genetic counselling should be offered, and children with a parent who has had a retinoblastoma should be assessed from infancy, shortly after birth. It is possible to detect the mutated gene by molecular techniques.

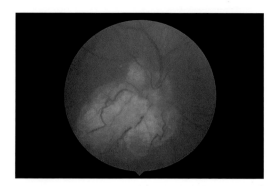

Figure 11.13 The clinical appearance of a retinal astrocytoma.

Prognosis

This depends on the extent of the disease at diagnosis. Overall the mortality of the condition is 15%. Unfortunately some 50% of children with the germinal mutation will develop a second primary tumour (e.g. an osteosarcoma of the femur) or a tumour related to treatment with radiotherapy.

Astrocytomas

These tumours of the retina and optic nerve (Fig. 11.13) are seen in patients with:
- tuberose sclerosis;
- neurofibromatosis (less commonly).

They appear as white berry-like lesions, are seldom symptomatic, and require no treatment. However, their identification may assist in the diagnosis of important systemic disease.

Choroidal tumours

Melanoma

Pigmented fundus lesions include:
- retinal pigment hypertrophy;
- areas of old chorioretinitis;
- choroidal naevi;
- the rarest cause, a malignant melanoma.

Uveal melanomas have an incidence of 6 per 1 000 000 per year in white adults. It is seen very much more commonly in white than in non-white races. It usually presents from middle age onwards (40–70 years). Malignant melanoma may also

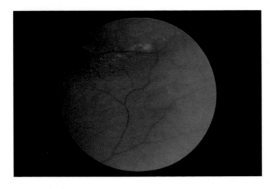

Figure 11.14 The clinical appearance of a choroidal melanoma.

be seen in the ciliary body and iris, but by far the greatest number (80%) are found in the choroid.

Symptoms

The presence of a melanoma may be detected as a coincidental finding during ocular examination (Fig. 11.14). Advanced cases may present with a visual field defect or loss of acuity. If situated in the anterior part of the choroid the enlarging tumour may cause shallowing of the anterior chamber, resulting in secondary angle closure glaucoma. In the UK it is unusual for the tumour to be so advanced that it results in visible destruction of the eye.

Signs

A raised, usually pigmented, lesion is visible at the back of the eye; this may be associated with an area of retinal detachment. The optic nerve may be involved.

Investigations

The patient is investigated for systemic spread, although this is less usual than in malignant melanoma of the skin. An ultrasound of the eye is useful in determining the size of the tumour and can be used both for quantitative assessment and in detecting tumour growth over time.

Treatment

A number of therapies are available. The treatment used depends on the size and location of the tumour. Large tumours that have reduced vision, or that are close to the optic nerve, usually require removal of the eye (enucleation). Smaller tumours can be treated by:

- local excision;
- local radiation applied to the lesion by an overlying radioactive plaque;
- proton beam irradiation.

Prognosis

This depends very much on the type of tumour (some are more rapidly growing than others) and its location (tumours involving the sclera and optic nerve carry a poorer prognosis). The existence of metastatic lesions at the time of diagnosis carries a poor prognosis. Some tumours are very slow-growing and have an excellent prognosis. Others, which extend into the optic nerve or through the sclera, are more malignant and result in secondary spread.

Metastatic tumours

These account for the greater part of ocular malignant disease. In women the commonest site of spread is from the breast; in men the commonest source is the lung. Symptoms and signs depend on their location in the eye. They appear as a whitish lesion with little elevation, and may be multiple. Treatment is usually by external beam radiotherapy.

Key points

- A curtain-like partial loss of vision suggests a retinal detachment and requires urgent ophthalmic assessment.
- Distortion of vision is a sign of macular disease.
- Age-related macular degeneration results in loss of acuity but never total loss of vision.
- Children with a white pupil require urgent ophthalmic investigation.

Multiple choice questions

1. Match the symptoms with the likely abnormal part of the retina

a Distortion of vision (metamorphopsia).

b Loss of superior visual field.

c Difficulty seeing at night.

   i The inferior half of the retina.

   ii The macula.

   iii The rods.

   iv The cones.

2. Age-related macular degeneration

a Is the commonest cause of irreversible visual loss in the developed world.

b Is associated with disease of the retinal pigment epithelium.

c May be associated with the growth of blood vessels beneath the retina.

d Is caused by a hole forming at the macula.

e Is commonly treated with surgery.

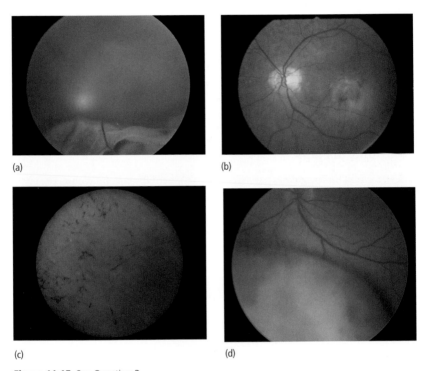

(a)

(b)

(c)

(d)

Figure 11.15 See Question 3.

3. Match the pictures (Fig. 11.15) with the diagnoses

a Age related macular degeneration (AMD).

b Macular hole.

c Retinal detachment.

d Melanoma.

e Retinitis pigmentosa.

4. Macular oedema

a Relates to the accumulation of fluid within the macula.

b Causes blurring of vision.

c May be seen following intraocular surgery.
d Is usually associated with the growth of abnormal vessels in the retina.
e Can be treated with steroids.

5. A patient presents with a history of three days of floaters, flashing lights and then a dense, curtain-like field loss.
a The most likely diagnosis is a retinal vein occlusion.
b The most likely diagnosis is a retinal detachment.
c The most likely diagnosis is a posterior vitreous detachment.
d The patient needs urgent referral to an eye unit.
e The vision will settle with no intervention.

6. A one-year-old child presents with a squint. The doctor notices that the red reflex appears white.
a A white red reflex is a normal finding in a child of this age.
b The child may have a retinoblastoma.
c The child has albinism.
d Urgent referral is required.
e The other eye needs to be assessed.

Answers

1. Match the symptoms with the likely abnormal part of the retina.
a The macula.
b The inferior half of the retina.
c The rods.

2. Age-related macular degeneration
a True.
b True.
c True.
d False. This is a separate condition, a macular hole.
e False. It is most often untreatable. In some patients with wet macular degeneration laser treatment, intravitreal anti-VEGF treatment, and rarely retinal surgery, may prevent visual deterioration.

3. Match the pictures (Fig. 11.15) with the diagnoses
a A retinal detachment.
b Age-related macular degeneration (AMD).
c Retinitis pigmentosa.
d Melanoma.

4. Macular oedema

a True.

b True.

c True.

d False.

e True.

5. A patient presents with a history of three days of floaters, flashing lights and then a dense, curtain-like field loss.

a False.

b True.

c False. Although the symptoms of flashes and floaters suggest a posterior vitreous detachment, the field loss indicates that a hole has been torn in the retina, causing a retinal detachment.

d True.

e False. The patient will lose the vision in the eye if urgent treatment is not given.

6. A one-year-old child presents with a squint. The doctor notices that the red reflex appears white.

a False. Leucocoria always requires urgent examination and investigation. Retinoblastoma is a life-threatening possibility.

b True.

c False. The red reflex would be present.

d True.

e True. Retinoblastoma may be bilateral.

Chapter 12

Retinal vascular disease

Learning objectives

To understand:
- The features of retinal vascular disease.
- The classification and treatment of diabetic retinopathy.
- The symptoms, signs and complications of retinal arterial and venous occlusion.
- The causes, features and treatment of retinopathy of prematurity.

Introduction

The eye is an organ in which much of the microcirculation is readily visualized. Vascular disease affecting the eye can thus be seen directly. Furthermore the eye provides important clues about pathological vascular changes in the rest of the body.

Signs of retinal vascular disease

The signs of retinal vascular disease (Figs 12.1, 12.2) result from two changes to the retinal capillary microcirculation:

1 vascular leakage;
2 vascular occlusion.

Leakage from the microcirculation

This results in:
- *Haemorrhages* caused by leakage of blood from damaged vessels.
- *Oedema* of the retina, the result of fluid leakage from damaged vessels.

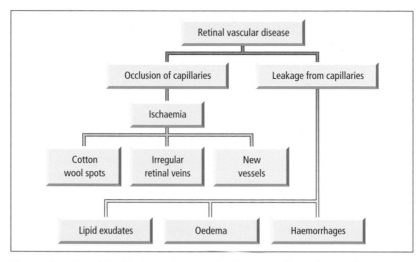

Figure 12.1 The building blocks of retinal vascular disease. Capillary leakage and acclusion often occur together.

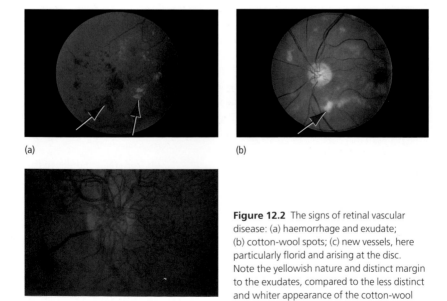

(a)

(b)

(c)

Figure 12.2 The signs of retinal vascular disease: (a) haemorrhage and exudate; (b) cotton-wool spots; (c) new vessels, here particularly florid and arising at the disc. Note the yellowish nature and distinct margin to the exudates, compared to the less distinct and whiter appearance of the cotton-wool spots.

Classification of diseases affecting the ocular circulation

Diabetic retinopathy
Central retinal artery occlusion
Branch retinal artery occlusion
Central retinal vein occlusion
Branch retinal vein occlusion
Hypertensive retinopathy
Retinopathy of prematurity
Sickle cell retinopathy
Abnormal retinal blood vessels

- *Exudates* formed by lipids, lipoprotein and lipid-containing macrophages. These are yellow in colour, with well-defined margins.

Occlusion of the microcirculation

This results in:
- *Cotton-wool spots* (previously termed *soft exudates*), fluffy white focal lesions with indistinct margins. They occur at the margins of an ischaemic retinal infarct due to obstruction of axoplasmic flow and build-up of axonal debris in the nerve fibre layer of the retina. Their visibility depends on nerve fibre layer thickness, so they are readily seen close to the optic disc, where the nerve fibre layer is thick, and not in the periphery, where the nerve fibre layer is thin. They are white in colour because the accumulated axoplasmic particles scatter light, whereas the normal nerve fibre is transparent.
- *New vessels.* An ischaemic retina releases vasogenic factors (e.g. VEGF) which result in the growth of abnormal blood vessels and fibrous tissue onto the retinal surface and forwards into the vitreous. These intravitreal vessels are much more permeable than normal retinal vessels and their abnormal location predisposes them to break and bleed.

Diabetic retinopathy

Diabetes results from a defect in both insulin secretion and action, leading to hyperglycaemia.

Epidemiology

Diabetic eye disease is the commonest reason for blind registration in the UK, in the 30–65 age group.

Type I diabetes (eventual loss of insulin secretion, mostly in young people with associated HLA types) has a prevalence in the UK of 2 per 1000 under the age of 20. Onset is relatively acute and diabetic retinopathy begins to appear about five years after onset.

Type II diabetes occurs in a heterogeneous group of patients and shows familial aggregation. Patients usually retain some insulin secretion but develop resistance to the action of insulin. It occurs in an older age group and has a prevalence of 5–20 per 1000. Because type II diabetes may be present for several years prior to diagnosis, retinopathy may be found at presentation.

Diabetes is associated with the following ocular events:

• Retinopathy.

• Cataract: a rare 'snowflake' cataract in youth, and a greater frequency and earlier onset of age-related cataract.

• Glaucoma (e.g. rubeotic glaucoma, but an association with chronic open angle glaucoma is disputed).

• Extraocular muscle palsy due to microvascular disease of the third, fourth or sixth cranial nerves.

Pathology

Factors thought to be important in the development of diabetic retinopathy include:

• Duration of diabetes: 80% have retinopathy after 20 years of disease.

• Diabetic control.

• Coexisting diseases, particularly hypertension.

• Smoking.

The development of retinopathy may also be accelerated by pregnancy, and patients require careful screening.

Retinal damage results from damage to the circulation. Pathological studies show:

• A decrease in the number of pericytes surrounding the capillary endothelium.

• Development of microaneurysms on the capillary network, which allow plasma to leak out into the retina.

• Patchy closure of the capillary net, resulting in areas of ischaemic retina and the development of arteriovenous shunts.

History

Diabetic retinopathy should be diagnosed before it is symptomatic. All diabetics should have fundoscopy performed at least yearly. Screening for sight-threatening retinopathy (maculopathy and proliferative retinopathy) should begin by five years after diagnosis in patients with type I disease, and from the time of presenta-

Table 12.1 The classification of diabetic retinopathy (note that diabetic maculopathy may coexist with other stages in the classification).

Stage	Description
No retinopathy	There are no abnormal signs present on the retina. *Vision normal.*
Background	Signs of microvascular leakage (haemorrhage and exudates) away from the macula. *Vision normal.*
Maculopathy	Exudates and haemorrhages within the macula region, and/or evidence of retinal oedema, and/or evidence of retinal ischaemia. *Vision is reduced; sight-threatening.*
Preproliferative	Evidence of occlusion (cotton-wool spots). The veins become irregular and may show loops. *Vision normal.*
Proliferative	The occlusive changes have led to the release of a vasoproliferative substance from the retina, resulting in the growth of new vessels either on the disc (NVD) or elsewhere on the retina (NVE). *Vision normal; sight-threatening.*
Advanced	The proliferative changes may result in bleeding into the vitreous or between the vitreous and the retina. The neuro retina may also be pulled from its overlying pigment epithelium by a fibrous proliferation associated with the growth of the new vessels. *Vision is reduced, often acutely, with vitreous haemorrhage; sight-threatening.*

tion in type II disease. Since its time of onset is unknown. Visual acuity may be reduced gradually by a maculopathy, or suddenly by a vitreous haemorrhage.

Examination

The building blocks of the disease are those of leakage and microvascular occlusion, discussed earlier. The classification of retinopathy is shown in Table 12.1.

Treatment

All diabetic patients should be screened for signs of retinopathy (Fig. 12.3). In the UK a screening programme using digital retinal photographs is being used to review patients on a yearly basis.

Patients with a maculopathy, preproliferative or proliferative retinopathy or worse require referral to an ophthalmologist. Any patient with unexplained visual loss should also be referred. The mainstay of treatment for sight-threatening diabetic retinopathy is laser therapy. A fluorescein angiogram may be performed in some patients to assess the degree of retinal ischaemia and to pinpoint areas of leakage both from microaneurysms and from new vessels.

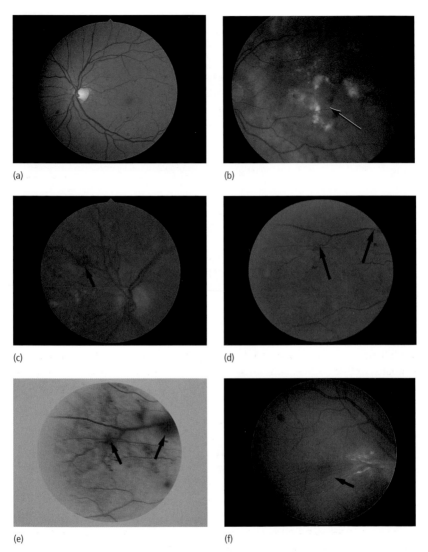

(a)

(b)

(c)

(d)

(e)

(f)

Figure 12.3 The signs of diabetic eye disease. (a) Background diabetic retinopathy. (b) Diabetic maculopathy: note the circinate exudate temporal to the macula. (c) Preproliferative retinopathy with a venous loop. (d, e) Proliferative retinopathy: new vessels have formed on the retina, their presence demonstrated by leakage of fluorescein (hyperfluorescence) on the fluorescein angiogram; closure of some of the retinal capillary network is demonstrated by its failure to fill with fluorescein. (f) Advanced diabetic retinopathy: the neovascularization has caused a traction retinal detachment.

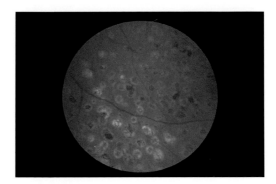

Figure 12.4 Typical appearance of retinal laser burns.

Diabetic retinopathy: clinical observations

- Younger patients are more likely to develop proliferative disease.
- Older patients more commonly develop a maculopathy, but because type II disease is more common, it is also an important cause of proliferative disease.

Laser treatment of both the maculopathy and new vessels can be performed on an outpatient basis.

- Diabetic maculopathy is treated by aiming the laser at the points of leakage. The exudate is often seen to be in a circinate pattern, with the focus of leakage or microaneurysm in the middle. If treatment is effective, the retinal oedema and exudate will resorb, although this may take some months.
- Optic disc and retinal new vessels are treated with scattered laser burns to the entire retina, leaving an untreated area around the macula and optic disc (Fig. 12.4). The laser treatment eliminates ischaemic retina, thus preventing the release of vasoproliferative factors. This results in the regression of the new vessels and prevents the development of advanced retinopathy.

The development of vitreous haemorrhage which does not clear after a few weeks, or fibrous traction on the retina causing detachment from the overlying pigment epithelium (traction retinal detachment), may require surgical treatment. A vitrectomy is performed to remove the vitreous gel and blood and to repair any of the detached retina.

Prognosis

Although laser and surgical treatments have greatly improved the prognosis of patients with diabetic retinopathy, the disease may still progress and cause severe visual loss in some patients.

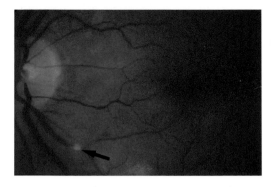

Figure 12.5 The clinical appearance of a cholesterol embolus (arrow). They appear to sparkle when viewed with a direct ophthalmoscope.

Arterial occlusion

Pathogenesis

Central and branch retinal artery occlusions are usually embolic in origin. Three types of emboli are recognized:

1 *fibrin-platelet* emboli, commonly from diseased carotid arteries;
2 *cholesterol* emboli, commonly from diseased carotid arteries (Fig. 12.5);
3 *calcific* emboli, from diseased heart valves.

History

The patient complains of a sudden painless loss of all or part of the vision. Fibrin-platelet emboli typically cause a fleeting loss of vision as the emboli pass through the retinal circulation (*amaurosis fugax*). This may last for some minutes, and then it clears. Cholesterol and calcific emboli may result in permanent obstruction with no recovery in vision (they may also be seen in the retinal vessels of asymptomatic individuals). A central retinal artery obstruction is frequently caused by an embolus, although as it lodges further back in the arterial tree behind the optic nerve head it cannot be seen.

In young patients, transient loss of vision may be caused by migraine.

Signs

Occasionally, a series of white platelet emboli can be seen passing rapidly through a vessel; more often a bright yellow, reflective cholesterol embolus is noted occluding an arterial branch point. The acutely affected retina is swollen and white (*oedematous*), while the fovea is red (*cherry-red spot*) because the choroid can be seen through the thin retina of the fovea. After several weeks the disc becomes pale (*atrophic*) and the arterioles attenuated. The condition may also occasionally be caused by vasculitis, such as giant cell arteritis (see Chapter 14).

Investigation

Patients require a careful vascular work-up, since disease in the eye may reflect systemic vascular disease. A search for carotid artery disease should be made by assessing the strength of carotid pulsation and listening for bruits. Ischaemic heart disease, peripheral claudication and hypertension may also be present.

A carotid endarterectomy may be indicated to prevent the possibility of a cerebral embolus if a stenosis of the carotid artery greater than 75% is present. Doppler ultrasound allows non-invasive imaging of both the carotid and vertebral arteries to detect such a stenosis.

Treatment

Acute treatment of central and branch artery occlusions is aimed at dilating the arteriole to permit the embolus to pass more distally and limit the damage. Results are usually disappointing, although a trial is worthwhile if the patient is seen within 24 hours of onset of the obstruction. The patient is referred to an eye unit, where the following measures may be tried:

- lowering the intraocular pressure with intravenous acetazolamide;
- ocular massage;
- paracentesis (a needle is inserted into the anterior chamber to release aqueous and lower the intraocular pressure rapidly);
- asking the patient to rebreathe into a paper bag firmly applied around the mouth and nose to use the vasodilatatory effect of raised carbon dioxide levels.

Prognosis

Full visual recovery occurs with amaurosis fugax, but more prolonged arterial occlusion results in severe, unrecoverable visual loss.

Venous occlusion

Pathogenesis

Central retinal vein occlusion (CRVO) may result from:
- abnormality of the blood itself (the hyperviscosity syndromes and abnormalities in coagulation);

- an abnormality of the venous wall (inflammation);
- an increased ocular pressure.

History

The patient complains of a sudden partial or complete loss of vision, although onset may be less acute than that of arterial occlusion.

Signs

These contrast markedly with those of arterial occlusion (Fig. 12.6). There is marked haemorrhage and great tortuosity and swelling of the veins. The optic disc appears swollen. Branch retinal vein occlusion may originate at the crossing point of an arteriole and a vein where the arteriole has been affected by arteriosclerosis associated with hypertension (A/V nipping).

Subsequently:
- Abnormal new vessels may grow on the retina and optic disc, causing vitreous haemorrhage. This happens if the retina has become ischaemic as a result of the vein occlusion (an ischaemic retinal vein occlusion).
- In ischaemic retinal vein occlusion abnormal new vessels may grow on the iris, causing rubeotic glaucoma.

Investigation

Investigation of a CRVO includes vascular and haematological work-up to exclude increased blood viscosity. Central retinal vein occlusion is also associated with raised ocular pressure, diabetes and hypertension and smoking.

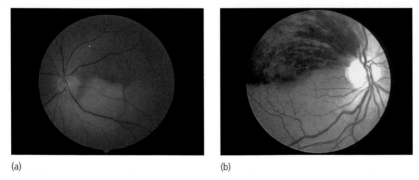

(a) (b)

Figure 12.6 The contrast between: (a) an inferior branch retinal artery occlusion (note the white appearance of the affected retina) and (b) a superior branch vein occlusion.

Treatment

Retinal laser treatment is given if the retina is ischaemic, to prevent the development of retinal and iris new vessels (see glaucoma, Chapter 10). Laser treatment may improve vision in some patients with a branch retinal vein occlusion by reducing macular oedema which may also be treated with intravitreal therapy.

Prognosis

The vision is usually severely affected in central, and often in branch, vein occlusion and usually does not improve. Younger patients may fare better, and there may well be some visual improvement.

Arteriosclerosis and hypertension

Arteriosclerosis can be visualized in the eye as an attenuation of the retinal arterial vessels (sometimes referred to as *copper* and *silver wiring*) and by the presence of *nipping* of the retinal vein where it is crossed by an arteriole. Hypertension in addition may cause focal arteriolar narrowing and a breakdown in the blood–retina barrier, resulting in the signs of vascular leakage (haemorrhage and exudate). These are particularly prominent if the hypertension is of renal origin. If severe, the retina may also demonstrate signs of capillary occlusion (cotton-wool spots). Very high blood pressure may, in addition, cause swelling of the optic nerve head as well as these other signs (*accelerated hypertension*; Fig. 12.7). The patient may complain of blurring of vision and of episodes of temporary visual loss, although severe retinopathy may also be asymptomatic.

Treatment of the hypertension results in the resolution of the retinal signs over some months. A rapid reduction of systemic blood pressure is avoided, because it may precipitate vascular occlusion.

Retinopathy of prematurity

Retinopathy of prematurity is a vascular response of the retina occurring predominantly in low-birthweight premature infants exposed to oxygen therapy in the early weeks of life. It leads to a traction detachment of the retina and potentially to bilateral blindness.

Pathogenesis

There is an initial failure of normal retinal vascularization, followed by a phase of aggressive new vessel formation extending forward into the vitreous and causing traction detachment.

179

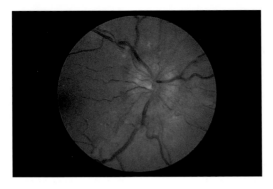

Figure 12.7 The fundus in malignant hypertension. The disc is swollen, and there are retinal haemorrhages and exudates.

Risk factors associated with retinopathy of prematurity include:

- gestation less than 32 weeks;
- birthweight below 1500 g;
- exposure to supplemental oxygen;
- apnoea;
- sepsis;
- duration of ventilation;
- blood transfusion;
- the presence of intraventricular haemorrhage;
- retinal light exposure.

The incidence of the condition in infants weighing less than 1500 g is between 34% and 60%.

Signs

The retinal appearance depends on the severity of the condition, but it includes:

- new vessels;
- the development of retinal haemorrhage;
- increased tortuosity and dilation of the retinal vessels.

In severe disease blindness can result from:

- bleeding into the vitreous;
- retinal detachment.

Treatment

At-risk infants are screened on a regular basis. The severe complications of the condition can be reduced by applying cryotherapy or laser to the avascular retina.

Sickle cell retinopathy

Patients with sickle cell haemoglobin C disease (SC disease) and sickle cell haemoglobin with thalassaemia (SThal) develop a severe form of retinopathy. This is unusual in homozygous sickle cell disease (SS), where the retinopathy is more confined. Signs include:

- tortuous veins;
- peripheral haemorrhages;
- capillary non-perfusion;
- pigmented spots on the retina;
- new vessel formation, classically in a 'sea fan' pattern, which may occur as a result of peripheral retinal artery occlusion.

New vessels may cause vitreous haemorrhage and traction retinal detachment. As with diabetes, this may require treatment with laser photocoagulation and vitrectomy.

Abnormal retinal blood vessels

Abnormalities of the retinal blood vessels may be seen in rare ocular diseases, associated with the development of massive exudate. They may also be an indication of systemic disorders, as in the retinal and optic disc angioma associated with the familial von Hippel–Lindau syndrome. Here the ocular condition may be associated with angioma in the brain and spinal cord. Patients and their relatives require repeated MRI screening.

Abnormalities of the blood

Clotting abnormalities may be responsible for occlusion of any blood vessel in the eye (e.g. a central retinal vein occlusion). Similarly, increased viscosity may also cause vessel occlusion. Leukaemia with a greatly raised white cell count may lead to the development of a haemorrhagic retinopathy in which the haemorrhages have white centres (*Roth spots*) (Fig. 12.8). These may also be a feature of bacterial endocarditis and autoimmune diseases associated with vasculitis.

Key points

- Premature infants require screening for retinopathy of prematurity.
- Diabetics require regular screening for sight-threatening retinopathy.

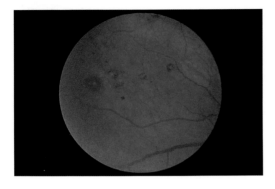

Figure 12.8 White-centred haemorrhages.

Multiple choice questions

1. Assign each of these signs of retinal vascular disease to either *leakage* or *occlusion*

a Haemorrhage.

b New vessels.

c Cotton-wool spot.

d Exudate.

e Oedema.

2. A central retinal vein occlusion

a Does not usually cause loss of vision.

b May be associated with the formation of new vessels.

c May be a cause of rubeotic glaucoma.

d May be associated with hypertension.

e Produces few abnormal signs in the retina.

3. Diabetic retinopathy

a Is seen in 80% of patients who have had diabetes for 20 years.

b Control of systemic hypertension is important in reducing the severity of the retinopathy.

c The number of pericytes around the capillaries is increased.

d Vitreous haemorrhage is associated with the formation of new vessels on the retina or optic nerve head.

e Circinate patterns of exudates are treated with scattered laser.

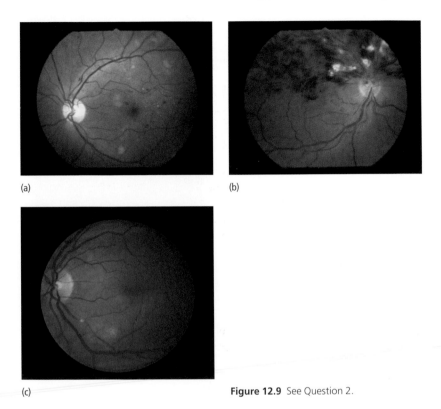

(a)

(b)

(c)   **Figure 12.9** See Question 2.

4. Match the pictures (Fig. 12.9) with the diagnoses
  i Diabetic retinopathy.
  ii Sickle cell retinopathy.
  iii Bacterial endocarditis.
  iv Retinal vein occlusion.
  v Retinopathy of prematurity.
  vi Retinal artery occlusion.
  vii Retinal arteriole embolus.

5. Retinopathy of prematurity
a Is caused by a failure of normal retinal vascularization.
b Is most commonly seen in babies with a low birthweight.
c Is less commonly seen in babies exposed to supplementary oxygen.
d New vessels and haemorrhages may be seen in the retina.
e Retinal detachment may complicate the condition.

Answers

1. Assign each of these signs of retinal vascular disease to either *leakage* or *occlusion*
a Leakage.
b Occlusion.
c Occlusion.
d Leakage.
e Leakage.

2. A central retinal vein occlusion
a False. ·
b True.
c True.
d True.
e False. The retinal veins are swollen and tortuous and there are extensive retinal haemorrhages.

3. Diabetic retinopathy
a True.
b True.
c False. The number is decreased.
d True.
e False. The laser is applied to the site of leakage, at the centre of the circinate exudate.

4. Match the pictures (Fig. 12.9) with the diagnoses
a Diabetic retinopathy. Note the haemorrhages, exudates and more peripheral cotton-wool spots.
b Retinal vein occlusion. This is a hemi-retinal vein occlusion.
c Retinal arteriole embolus.

5. Retinopathy of prematurity
a True.
b True.
c False.
d True.
e True.

Chapter 13

The pupil and its responses

Learning objectives

To understand:
- The neurological pathways controlling pupillary size and responses.
- The causes of pupillary dysfunction.

Introduction

Movements of the pupil are controlled by the parasympathetic and sympathetic nervous systems. The pupils constrict (*miosis*) when the eye is illuminated (parasympathetic activation, sympathetic relaxation) and dilate (*mydriasis*) in the dark (sympathetic activation, parasympathetic relaxation). When the eyes focus on a near object, they converge and the pupils constrict (the *near response*). The pupils are normally equal in size but some 20% of people may have noticeably unequal pupils (*anisocoria*) with no associated disease.

The key to diagnosis of pupillary disorders is to:
- determine which pupil is abnormal;
- search for associated signs.

Disorders of the pupil may result from:
- ocular disease;
- disorders of the controlling neurological pathway;
- pharmacological action.

The parasympathetic fibres reach the eye through the third cranial nerve. The sympathetic pathway is shown in Fig. 13.1.

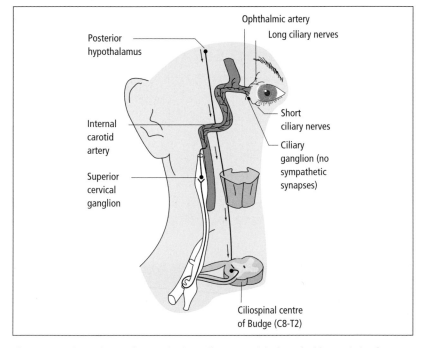

Figure 13.1 The pathway of sympathetic pupillary control. (Adapted with permission from Kanski, J. J. (1994) *Clinical Ophthalmology*. Butterworth–Heinemann, Oxford.)

Ocular causes of pupillary abnormality

Diseases of the eye which cause irregularity of the pupil and alter its reaction include:
• ocular inflammation, where posterior synechiae give the pupil an irregular appearance (see Chapter 9);
• the sequelae of intraocular surgery;
• blunt trauma to the eye, which may rupture the sphincter muscle, causing irregularity or fixed dilation (*traumatic mydriasis*).

Neurological causes of an abnormal pupil

Horner's syndrome

Interruption of the sympathetic pathway causes:
• A small pupil on the affected side (Fig. 13.2). This is more noticeable in the dark, when the fellow, normal pupil, dilates more than the affected pupil.
• A slight ptosis on the affected side.

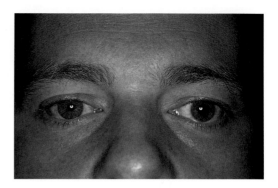

Figure 13.2 A right ptosis and miosis in Horner's syndrome.

• Lack of sweating on the affected side if the sympathetic pathway is affected proximal to the base of the skull affecting fibres travelling with the branches of the external carotid.

• An apparent recession of the globe into the orbit.

Because of its extended course the sympathetic pathway may be affected by a multitude of pathologies. Examples include:

• Syringomyelia, a cavity within the spinal cord sometimes extending into the medulla (syringobulbia). Typically it also causes wasting of the hand muscles and loss of sensation.

• Disease of the lung apex catches the cervical sympathetic chain (e.g. neoplasia). Involvement of the brachial plexus gives rise to pain and to T1 wasting of the small muscles of the hand in Pancoast's syndrome.

• Neck injury, disease or surgery.

• Cavernous sinus disease.

Horner's syndrome may also be congenital. Here the iris colour may be altered when compared to the fellow eye (*heterochromia*).

Light–near dissociation

In these pupillary abnormalities the reaction of the pupils to light is much less than to the near (accommodative) response. There is no condition in which the light reflex is intact but the near reflex is defective. A light–near dissociation is seen in diabetes and multiple sclerosis or may be caused by periaqueductal brainstem lesions (see below).

Relative afferent pupillary defect

A lesion of the optic nerve on one side blocks the afferent limb of the pupillary light reflex (see Chapter 2). The pupils are equal and of normal size, but the pupillary response to light on the affected side is reduced, while the near reflex is intact. This is an important test to perform in a patient suspected of having an optic nerve lesion, such as optic neuritis. It may also, however, be seen in severe disease of the retina. It is not seen with opacities of the cornea or lens.

Adie's pupil

This is a not uncommon cause of unequal pupil size (*anisocoria*). It affects young adults and is seen more commonly in females than in males (2 : 1). It is due to a ciliary ganglionitis which denervates the parasympathetic supply to the iris and ciliary body. Parasympathetic fibres which reinnervate the iris sphincter are those which were previously involved in accommodation. The sphincter is partially reinnervated, but the muscarinic receptors are supersensitive to cholinergic agonists.

Incomplete innervation of the sphincter causes the pupil to become:
• Enlarged.
• Poorly reactive to light. On the slit-lamp examination the pupil movement in response to light is seen as a worm-like (*vermiform*) contraction.
The result of muscarinic supersensitivity is that the pupil:
• Shows slow, sustained miosis on accommodation.
• Is supersensitive to dilute pilocarpine (0.1%) a diagnostic test.
The ability to accommodate is also impaired. The patient may complain of blurred vision when looking from a distant object to a near one, and vice versa. Systemically the disorder is associated with loss of tendon reflexes; there are no other neurological signs.

Argyll Robertson pupil

Classically seen in neurosyphilis: the pupils are bilaterally small and irregular. They do not react to light but do to accommodation. The iris stroma has a typical feathery appearance and loses its architectural detail.

Midbrain pupil

A lesion in the region of the pretectal nuclear complex disrupts retinotectal fibres but preserves the supranuclear accommodative pathway, causing mydriasis and light–near dissociation. This is usually seen as part of the *dorsal midbrain (Parinaud's) syndrome* (see Chapter 15).

Other causes of pupillary abnormality

In coma, both pupils may become miosed with preservation of the light reflex if a

Table 13.1 Drugs having a pharmacological effect on the pupil.

Agent	Action	Mechanism
Topical agents		
Dilates	Muscarinic blockade	Cyclopentolate
		Tropicamide
		Atropine (long-acting)
	Alpha-adrenergic agonist	Phenylephrine
		Adrenaline
		Dipivefrine
Constricts	Muscarinic agonist	Pilocarpine
Systemic agents		
Dilates	Muscarinic blockade	Atropine
	Alpha-adrenergic agonist	Adrenaline
Constricts	Local action and action on central nervous system	Morphine

pontine lesion is present, but remember that patients taking pilocarpine for glaucoma or receiving morphine also show bilateral miosis. Midbrain lesions cause loss of the light reflex with mid-point pupils. Coma associated with a unilateral expanding supratentorial mass, e.g. a haematoma, results in pressure on the third nerve and dilation of the pupil. Intrinsic third nerve lesions also cause a dilated pupil (see Chapter 15). The pupil may also be affected by drugs, both topical and systemic (Table 13.1).

Key points

- Take a good history to help exclude an ocular cause for the pupillary changes and to see if a medical condition exists which may contribute to the pupillary problem.
- Determine whether it is the small or the large pupil that is abnormal.
- Search for associated signs that may help make a diagnosis.

Multiple choice questions

1. Pathological miosis is seen in

a Horner's syndrome.

b Third nerve palsy.

c Argyll Robertson pupil.

d Coma.

e Systemic and topical atropine treatment.

2. Horner's syndrome may be seen in

a Syringomyelia.

b Lung neoplasia.

c Cavernous sinus disease.

d Myasthenia gravis.

e Carotid artery dissection.

3. Light–near dissociation

a The reaction of the pupils is greater to light than accommodation.

b May be seen in diabetes.

c Is seen in Horner's syndrome.

d Is seen in patients with an Argyll Robertson pupil.

e Is seen following administration of tropicamide drops.

4. Match the drop to its action: *dilates* **(mydriasis) or** *constricts* **(miosis)**

a Cyclopentolate.

b Atropine.

c Pilocarpine.

d Tropicamide.

e Phenylephrine.

Answers

1. Pathological miosis is seen in

a True.

b False.

c True.

d True.

e False.

2. Horner's syndrome may be seen in

a True.

b True. An apical lung tumour may catch the cervical sympathetic trunk as it leaves the inferior cervical ganglion.

c True.

d False. This may cause a ptosis but does not affect the pupil.

e True. This is a cause of a painful Horner's syndrome.

3. Light–near dissociation

a False. It is the other way round: the pupils react poorly to light.

b True.

c False. The pupil is smaller but reacts normally to light and accommodation.

d True.

e False. The pupil is dilated and unreactive to both stimuli.

4. Match the drop to its action

a Dilates.

b Dilates.

c Constricts.

d Dilates.

e Dilates.

Chapter 14

The visual pathway

Learning objectives

To understand:
- The basic anatomy of the visual pathway.
- The field defects produced by lesions at different points along the visual pathway.
- The causes, symptoms and signs associated with a swollen optic disc.
- The symptoms, signs, treatment and complications of giant cell arteritis.

Introduction

The innermost layer of the retina consists of the nerve fibres originating from the retinal ganglion cells. These fibres collect together at the optic nerve head, and form the optic nerve (see Chapter 1). The subsequent course of the visual pathway is shown in Fig. 14.1. Diagnosis and location of disease of the optic pathways is greatly aided by study of the differing field defects produced.

The optic nerve

The normal optic nerve head has distinct margins, a pinkish rim and usually a white central cup. The central retinal artery and vein enter the globe slightly nasally in the optic nerve head (optic disc). The optic disc may be involved in many disorders but has a limited repertoire of responses. Ophthalmoscopically it may become swollen, or it may become pale.

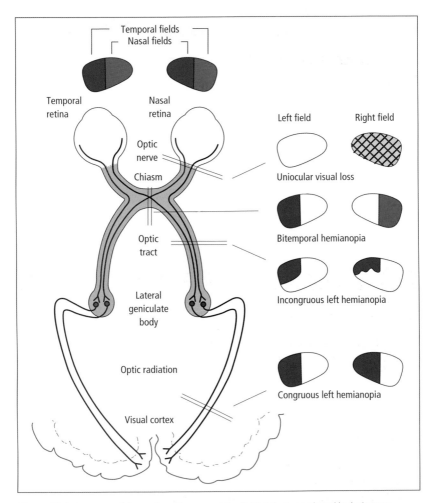

Figure 14.1 Anatomy of the optic pathway and the field defects produced by lesions at different sites.

The swollen optic disc

The swollen disc (Fig. 14.2) is an important and often worrying sign. *Papilloedema* is the term given to disc swelling associated with raised intracranial pressure, accelerated hypertension and optic disc ischaemia. Optic neuritis affecting the nerve head (*papillitis*) has a similar appearance. Visual loss always occurs with optic neuritis but is uncommon with the papilloedema of hypertension and raised intraacranial pressure; it is, however, a feature of ischaemic papilloedema.

193

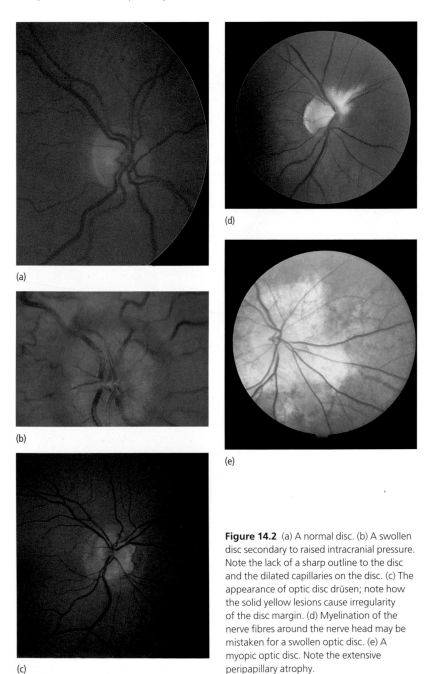

(a)

(b)

(c)

(d)

(e)

Figure 14.2 (a) A normal disc. (b) A swollen disc secondary to raised intracranial pressure. Note the lack of a sharp outline to the disc and the dilated capillaries on the disc. (c) The appearance of optic disc drüsen; note how the solid yellow lesions cause irregularity of the disc margin. (d) Myelination of the nerve fibres around the nerve head may be mistaken for a swollen optic disc. (e) A myopic optic disc. Note the extensive peripapillary atrophy.

Table 14.1 Causes of a swollen optic disc.

Condition	Distinguishing features
Raised intracranial pressure	Vision and field usually normal save for large blind spot. Obscurations (short episodes of visual loss usually on changing posture). Field may be contracted in chronic disease. Colour vision normal. No RAPD. No spontaneous venous pulsation of the vein at the disc (but some people with normal intracranial pressure do not have this). Dilated capillaries and haemorrhages on disc. Other symptoms and signs of raised intracranial pressure.
Space-occupying lesions of the optic nerve head	Various solid or infiltrative lesions at the nerve head, e.g. optic disc drüsen (calcified axonal material), gliomas, sarcoidosis and leukaemia, may produce disc swelling. These may be associated with reduced vision and field defects.
Papillitis (optic neuritis affecting the optic nerve head)	A swollen optic disc. Exudates around the macula may occasionally be seen. Vision is profoundly reduced. Colour vision is abnormal. RAPD present. A central field defect is present.
Accelerated (malignant) hypertension (see Chapter 12)	Reduced vision, haemorrhagic disc swelling. Retinal haemorrhages, exudates and cotton-wool spots away from the nerve head. Check blood pressure!
Ischaemic optic neuropathy	Sudden visual loss, field defect. Colour vision may be normal. RAPD may be present. Spontaneous venous pulsation at the optic disc may be present. May be sectorial swelling only. Haemorrhages on disc and disc margin. Cotton-wool spots may be seen around disc, particularly if caused by giant cell arteritis.
Central retinal vein occlusion (see Chapter 12)	Sudden marked visual loss, tortuous veins, gross retinal haemorrhage.

Apparent disc swelling must be distinguished from pseudopapilloedema such as optic nervehead drüsen, myelinated nerve fibres and the peripapillary atrophy of high myopia. RAPD, relative afferent pupillary defect; see Chapter 2.

The differential diagnosis of disc swelling is shown in Table 14.1. Some normal optic nerve heads may appear to be swollen, due a crowding of nerve fibres entering the disc. This is termed *pseudopapilloedema* and occurs particularly in small, hypermetropic eyes where the nerve entry site is reduced in size. Note also that *myelinated nerve fibres* occurring on the nerve head may be mistaken for optic disc swelling. These are a developmental variant in which the normally unmyelinated retinal nerve fibre layer is partly myelinated, giving it a feathery, white appearance. In high myopia the optic disc may be surrounded by an atrophic area (*peripapillary atrophy*), which may be confused with disc swelling.

Papilloedema due to raised intracranial pressure

History

The crucial feature of disc swelling due to raised intracranial pressure is that acutely there is rarely an associated visual loss, although some patients may develop fleeting visual loss lasting seconds when they alter posture (*obscurations* of vision). Other features of raised intracranial pressure may be present, including:

- headache, worse on waking and made worse by coughing;
- nausea, retching;
- diplopia (double vision), usually due to a sixth nerve palsy;
- neurological symptoms, if the raised pressure is due to a cranial space-occupying lesion;
- a history of head trauma suggesting a subdural haemorrhage.

Signs

- The optic disc is swollen, its edges are blurred, and the superficial capillaries are dilated and thus abnormally prominent. There is no spontaneous venous pulsation of the central retinal vein (5–20% of those with normal nerve heads have no spontaneous pulsation, but venous collapse at the nerve/head can be induced by light pressure on the globe.).
- A large blind spot will be found on visual field testing, corresponding to the swollen nerve head. In chronic papilloedema the field may become constricted. A field defect may, however, be caused by the space-occupying lesion causing the papilloedema.
- Abnormal neurological signs may indicate the site of a space-occupying lesion.

Investigation

CT and MRI scanning will identify any space-occupying lesion or enlargement of the ventricles. Following neurological consultation (and normally after a scan) a lumbar puncture will enable intracranial pressure to be measured.

Treatment

Intracranial pressure may be elevated and disc swelling present with no evidence of intracranial abnormality and no dilation of the ventricles on the scan. This is termed *benign intracranial hypertension* and usually presents in overweight women in the second and third decades. It may also be caused by exposure to certain drugs such as the contraceptive pill and tetracyclines. Patients complain of headache and may have obscurations of vision and sixth nerve palsies. No other neurological problems are present. Although acute permanent visual loss is not a feature of papilloedema, if the nerve remains swollen for several weeks there will be a progressive contraction of the visual field. It is thus important to reduce intracranial pressure. This may be achieved:

- with medications such as oral acetazolamide;
- through ventriculoperitoneal shunting;
- through optic nerve decompression, where a small hole is made in the sheath surrounding the optic nerve to allow the drainage of CSF and reduce the pressure of CSF around the anterior optic nerve.

Space-occupying lesions (i.e. tumours and haemorrhage) and hydrocephalus require neurosurgical management.

Optic neuritis

Inflammation or demyelination of the optic nerve results in optic neuritis (termed *papillitis* if the optic nerve head is affected and *retrobulbar neuritis* if the optic nerve is affected more posteriorly).

History

There is:
- An acute loss of vision that may progress over a few days and then slowly improve.
- Pain on eye movement in retrobulbar neuritis because rectus contraction pulls on the optic nerve sheath.
- A preceding history of viral illness in some cases. Between 40% and 70% of patients with optic neuritis will have or develop other neurological symptoms to suggest a diagnosis of demyelination (multiple sclerosis).

Examination

This reveals:
- reduced visual acuity;
- reduced colour vision;
- relative afferent pupillary defect (RAPD) (see Chapter 2);
- central scotoma on field testing;
- a normal disc in retrobulbar neuritis; a swollen disc in papillitis.

Treatment

An MRI scan will help to identify additional 'silent' plaques of demyelination, but the patient must be suitably counselled before a scan is performed. The diagnosis of multiple sclerosis is essentially a clinical one, and the patient may not wish to have the presence of other possible plaques confirmed with a scan. There may be a role for steroid treatment to speed up visual recovery.

Prognosis

Vision slowly recovers over several weeks, although often it is not quite as good as before the attack. Repeated episodes may lead to optic atrophy and a decline in vision. Very occasionally in atypical cases vision may not recover.

Ischaemic optic neuropathy

Pathogenesis

The anterior optic nerve may become ischaemic if the posterior ciliary vessels are compromised as a result of degenerative vaso-occlusive or vasculitic disease of the arterioles (see Chapter 1). This results in an *anterior ischaemic optic neuropathy*.

Symptoms

The patient complains of a sudden loss of vision or visual field, often on waking since vascular perfusion to the eye is decreased during sleep. If accompanied by pain or scalp tenderness the diagnosis of *giant cell arteritis* must never be forgotten. Ischaemic optic neuropathy is the usual cause of blindness in the disease.

Giant cell arteritis

This is an autoimmune vasculitis occurring in patients generally over the age of 60. It affects arteries with an internal elastic lamina. It may present with any combination of:

- sudden loss of vision;
- scalp tenderness (e.g. on combing);
- pain on chewing (*jaw claudication*);
- shoulder pain;
- malaise.

Signs

There is usually (Fig. 14.3):

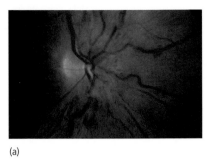

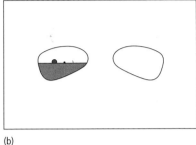

(a)   (b)

Figure 14.3 (a) The clinical appearance of the optic disc and (b) one form of field defect (altitudinal) seen in ischaemic optic neuropathy.

- A reduction in visual acuity.
- A field defect, typically an absence of the lower or upper half of the visual field.
- A swollen and haemorrhagic disc with normal retina and retinal vessels (remember the blood supply to the anterior optic nerve and retina are different). In arteritic ischaemic optic neuropathy the disc may be pale.
- A small fellow disc with a small cup in non-arteritic disease.
- A tender temporal artery, a sign suggestive of giant cell arteritis.

Investigations

If giant cell arteritis is present the ESR and C-reactive protein are usually grossly elevated (eg 100 mm/hr) (although 1 in 10 patients with giant cell arteritis have a normal ESR). Temporal artery biopsy is often helpful, but again may not lead to a diagnosis, particularly if only a small specimen is examined, because the disease may skip a length of the artery. Giant cell arteritis can also present as a central retinal artery occlusion when the vessel is affected secondarily to arteritis of the ophthalmic artery.

Investigation of the patient with non-arteritic ischaemic optic neuropathy includes:
- a full blood count to exclude anaemia;
- blood pressure check;
- blood sugar check;
- ESR and C-reactive protein to check for giant cell arteritis.

Both hypertension and diabetes may be associated with the condition. It may also be seen in patients suffering acute blood loss, e.g. haematemesis, where it may occur some days after the acute bleed. Hypotensive episodes may also give rise to ischaemic optic neuropathy. Occasionally, clotting disorders or autoimmune disease may cause the condition.

Treatment

If giant cell arteritis is suspected, treatment must not be delayed while the diagnosis is confirmed. High-dose steroids must be given, intravenously and orally, and the dose tapered over the ensuing weeks according to both symptoms and the response of the ESR or C-reactive protein. The usual precautions must be taken, as with any patient on steroids, to exclude other medical conditions that might be unmasked or made worse by the steroids (e.g. tuberculosis, diabetes, hypertension and an increased susceptibility to infection). Steroids will not reverse the visual loss but can prevent the fellow eye being affected.

There is unfortunately no treatment for non-arteritic ischaemic optic neuropathy other than through the management of underlying conditions.

Prognosis

It is unusual for the vision to get progressively worse in non-arteritic ischaemic optic neuropathy, and the visual outcome in terms of both visual field and acuity is very variable. Vision does not recover once it has been lost. The second eye may rapidly become involved in patients with untreated giant cell arteritis. There is also a significant rate of involvement of the second eye in the non-arteritic form (40–50%).

Optic atrophy

A pale optic disc represents a loss of nerve fibres at the optic nerve head (Fig. 14.4, Table 14.2). The vision is usually reduced, and colour vision affected. On examination the usual vascularity of the disc is lost. Comparison of the two eyes is of

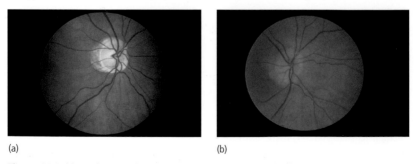

(a)   (b)

Figure 14.4 (a) A pale optic disc compared to (b) a normal optic disc.

Table 14.2 Causes of a pale optic disc.

Cause	Distinguishing features
Compression of the optic nerve	History of orbital or chiasmal disease. If sectorial, field loss may give a clue to the location of a compressive lesion.
Ischaemic optic neuropathy Retinal artery Retinal vein occlusion	A history of sudden (unilateral) visual loss in the past. The retinal vessels are attenuated.
Glaucoma (see Chapter 10)	The optic disc is pathologically cupped.
Optic neuritis	There may be a history of previous loss of vision. Symptoms and signs compatible with multiple sclerosis may be present.
Inherited optic nerve disease	Dominant and recessive optic neuropathy are associated with onset of blindness in the first few years of life. Leber's optic neuropathy results from an inheritable mutation of mitochondrial DNA. Leber's typically affects males in early adulthood. It is bilateral. The optic disc appears pale.
Inherited retinal disease	Retinal disease may result in optic disc pallor. It is, for example, a feature of rod–cone dystrophies and retinitis pigmentosa.
Toxic optic neuropathy	Optic neuropathy may follow chemical toxicity, for example heavy metals, toluene from glue-sniffing and some drugs (e.g. isoniazid used in the treatment of tuberculosis). Again, information should be sought in the history.
Tobacco/alcohol/nutritional vitamin amblyopia	Optic neuropathy here (where all three factors are often involved together) is due to a combination of vitamin deficiency (B_{12}) and cyanide toxicity.

great help in unilateral cases, as the contrast makes identification of pallor much easier. A relative afferent pupillary defect will also be present.

The chiasm

Compressive lesions at the chiasm produce a bitemporal hemianopia as the fibres representing the nasal retina (temporal field) are compressed as they cross in the

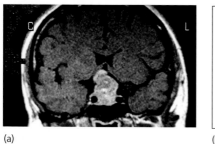
(a)

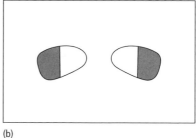
(b)

Figure 14.5 (a) The CT appearance of a pituitary tumour. (b) The bitemporal visual field loss produced.

centre of the chiasm. Patients may present with rather vague visual symptoms, for example:

• Missing objects in the periphery of the visual field.

• When testing vision with a Snellen chart patients may miss the temporal letters with each eye.

• The bitemporal field loss may cause difficulty in fusing images, causing the patient to complain of diplopia although eye movements are normal.

• There may be difficulty with tasks requiring stereopsis such as pouring water into a cup or threading a needle.

The most common lesion is a pituitary tumour (Fig. 14.5), and the patient should be asked for symptoms relating to hormonal disturbance. Treatment depends on the type of tumour found; some are amenable to medical therapy but many require surgical excision. A *meningioma* and *craniopharyngioma* may also cause chiasmal compression.

Optic tract, radiation and visual cortex

Lesions (usually either vascular or neoplastic) of the optic tract and radiation produce a *homonymous hemianopic field defect*, that is, loss confined to the right- or left-hand side of the field in both eyes (Fig. 14.6). This pattern of field loss results from the crossing of the fibres representing the nasal retina in the chiasm. If the extent of field loss is similar in both eyes a *congruous* defect is said to be present. This usually means that the defect has affected the optic radiation or cerebral cortex. Neoplasia more commonly affects the radiation in the anterior temporal lobe. The commonest cause of disease in the occipital cortex is a cerebrovascular accident. The visual loss is of rapid onset; a slower onset is suggestive of a space-occupying lesion.

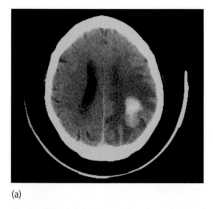
(a)

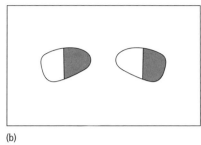
(b)

Figure 14.6 (a) A CT scan showing a left cortical infarct. (b) The complete congruous right homonymous hemianopia produced by the infarct.

<table>
<tr><td>Key points</td></tr>
</table>

- A bitemporal visual field defect suggests a pituitary lesion.
- There are several causes of a swollen optic disc; it is not just a sign of raised intracranial pressure.
- A pale optic disc may result from retinal disease.

Multiple choice questions

1. Match the field defect to the possible site of disease

a Unilateral central scotoma.
b Congruous left hemianopia.
c Bitemporal hemianopia.
d Unilateral superior field defect.
e Incongruous left hemianopia.
  i Optic chiasm.
  ii Visual cortex.
  iii Optic nerve.
  iv Optic tract.
  v Retina.

2. A swollen disc may be caused by

a Raised intraocular pressure.
b Raised intracranial pressure.
c Optic neuritis.
d Systemic hypertension.
e Central retinal artery occlusion.

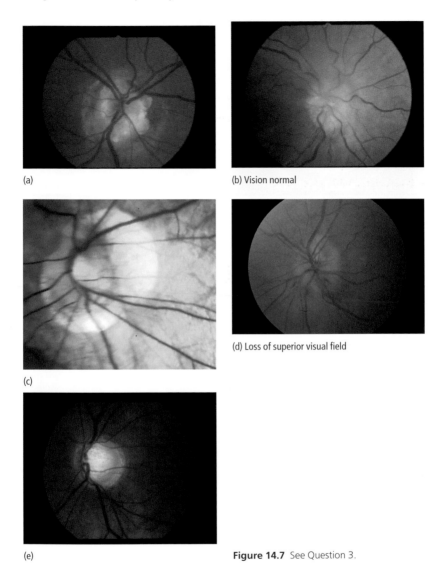

(a)

(b) Vision normal

(c)

(d) Loss of superior visual field

(e)

Figure 14.7 See Question 3.

3. Match the pictures (Fig. 14.7) to the most probable diagnosis

  i Optic disc drüsen.

  ii Glaucoma.

  iii Pituitary tumour.

  iv Ischaemic optic neuropathy.

  v Retinitis pigmentosa.

vi Myelination of the retinal nerve fibre layer.

vii Myopia.

viii Papilloedema.

ix Optic neuritis.

4. Optic neuritis

a Is associated with a sudden loss of vision that does not progress.

b Is painless.

c May be part of a systemic neurological disease.

d Vision rarely recovers.

e Is associated with a reduction in colour vision.

5. Ischaemic optic neuropathy

a Presents with an acute loss of vision.

b On examination the patient has a swollen disc.

c May be associated with scalp tenderness and jaw claudication.

d Should always be treated with steroids.

e May cause an altitudinal field defect.

6. Optic atrophy may be seen in

a Some retinal diseases.

b Compression of the optic nerve.

c Diseases of the visual cortex.

d Toxic eye disease.

e Poor nutrition.

Answers

1. Match the field defect to the possible site of disease

a Optic nerve or retina.

b Visual cortex.

c Optic chiasm.

d Retina or optic nerve.

e Optic tract.

2. A swollen disc may be caused by

a False. A chronic rise in pressure will produce pathological cupping of the optic disc.

b True.

c True. This is then called papillitis; but the optic nerve head appears normal in retrobulbar neuritis.

d True. But only in severe or accelerated hypertension.

e False. It is seen in a central retinal vein occlusion and in ischaemic optic neuropathy.

3. Match the pictures (Fig. 14.7) to the most probable diagnosis
a Optic disc drüsen.

b Papilloedema.

c Myopia.

d Ischaemic optic neuropathy.

e Glaucoma.

4. Optic neuritis
a False. The visual loss usually progresses over a couple of days.

b False. There may be pain on eye movement in retrobulbar neuritis.

c True. It may be due to demyelination and be part of multiple sclerosis.

d False. There is usually some degree of recovery.

e True. This is a useful test in assessing optic nerve disease.

5. Ischaemic optic neuropathy
a True.

b True.

c True. The condition may be a feature of giant cell arteritis. It is important to think of this in any senior patient, but there are also non-arteritic vascular causes.

d False. If it is associated with giant cell arteritis this is the immediate treatment. Non-arteritic disease does not respond to steroids.

e True.

6. Optic atrophy may be seen in
a True. It may be seen for example in retinitis pigmentosa.

b True.

c False. Disc pallor will only be seen in lesions anterior to the lateral geniculate body.

d True. e.g. tobacco–alcohol or ethambutol toxicity.

e True. An example is vitamin B_{12} deficiency.

Chapter 15

Eye movements and their disorders

Learning objectives

To understand:
- The actions and control of the six muscles moving the eye.
- The difference between non-paralytic and paralytic squint.
- What is meant by binocular single vision.
- The cause, investigation and treatment of non-paralytic squint.
- The symptoms, signs and treatment of paralytic squint.
- The importance of the differential diagnosis of third nerve palsy.
- Gaze palsy and nystagmus.

To be able to:
- Perform a cover test.

Introduction

Eye movements may be abnormal because there is:
- an abnormal position of the eyes;
- a reduced range of eye movement;
- an abnormality in the form of eye movement.

Anatomy and physiology

Each eye can be *abducted* (away from the nose) or *adducted* (towards the nose) or may look up (*elevation*) or down (*depression*). The cardinal positions of gaze for assessing a muscle palsy are: gaze right, left, up, down, and gaze to the right and left in the up and down positions.

Six extraocular muscles control eye movement. The medial and lateral recti bring about horizontal eye movements causing adduction and abduction respectively. The superior and inferior recti elevate and depress the eye in abduction. The superior oblique causes depression of the eye in the adducted position and the inferior oblique causes elevation in the adducted position. The vertical muscles all have additional, secondary, rotatory actions (intorsion and extorsion, circular movement of the eye).

Three cranial nerves supply these muscles (see Chapter 1), and their nuclei are found in the brainstem, together with pathways linking them with other brainstem nuclei (e.g. vestibular) and with gaze centres (horizontal gaze in the pons and vertical gaze in the midbrain). These coordinate the movements of both eyes.

Higher cortical centres control the speed with which the eyes follow a moving

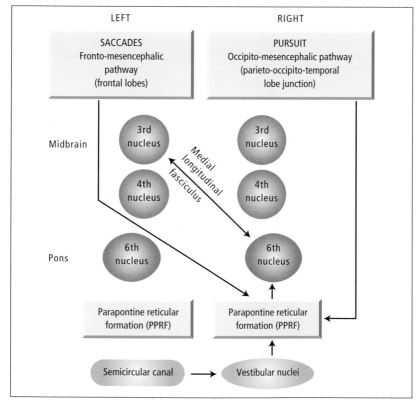

Figure 15.1 The connections of the nuclei and higher centres controlling horizontal eye movements. Saccade and pursuit pathways shown for right eye only.

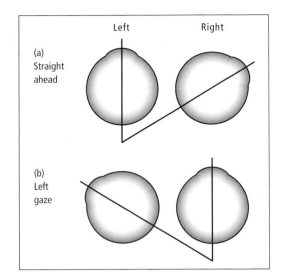

Figure 15.2 The pattern of eye movement seen in a non-paralytic squint. (a) The right eye is divergent in the primary position of gaze (looking straight ahead). (b) When the eyes look to the left the angle of deviation between the *visual axis* (a line passing through the point of fixation and the foveola) of the two eyes is unchanged.

target (*smooth pursuit*), and the rapid movements required to take up another position of gaze (*saccades*). These centres also influence the brainstem nuclei.

The linkage of the nuclei ensures that the eyes move together in a coordinated fashion (Fig. 15.1). For example, when looking to the right, the right lateral and left medial rectus are equally stimulated and are said to be *yoke muscles*. At the same time innervation of the antagonists which move the eyes to the left (the left lateral rectus and the right medial rectus) is inhibited.

Clinically, eye movement disorders are best described under four headings (which are not mutually exclusive):

1 In a *non-paralytic squint* the movements of both eyes are full (there is no paresis) but only one eye is directed towards the fixated target (Fig. 15.2). The angle of deviation is constant and unrelated to the direction of gaze. This is also termed a *concomitant squint*, and it is the common squint that is seen in childhood.

2 In a *paralytic squint* there is underaction of one or more of the eye muscles due to a nerve palsy, extraocular muscle disease or tethering of the globe. The size of the squint is dependent on the direction of gaze and thus, for a nerve palsy, is greatest in the *field of action* of the affected muscle (i.e. the direction in which the muscle would normally take the globe) (Fig. 15.3). This is also termed an *incomitant squint*.

3 In *gaze palsies* there is a disturbance of the supranuclear coordination of eye movements. Pursuit and saccadic eye movements may also be affected if the cortical pathways to the nuclei controlling eye movements are interrupted.

4 Disorders of the brainstem nuclei or vestibular input may also result in a form of oscillating eye movement termed *nystagmus*.

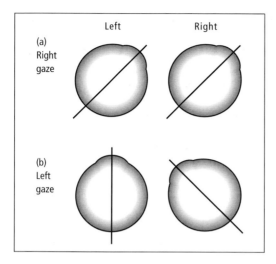

Figure 15.3 The pattern of eye movement seen in a left sixth nerve palsy with paralysis of the left lateral rectus. (a) The eyes are looking to the right, the visual axes are aligned, there is no deviation between the visual axes of the two eyes. (b) The eyes look to the left (the field of action of the left lateral rectus). The left lateral rectus is paralysed and thus the left eye is unable to move past the midline. Now there is a marked angle of deviation between the visual axes of the two eyes.

Non-paralytic squint

Binocular single vision

In the absence of a squint (*strabismus*), both eyes are directed towards the same object of regard. Their movements are coordinated so that the retinal images of an object fall on corresponding points of each retina. These images are fused centrally, so that they are interpreted by the brain as a single image. This is termed *binocular single vision* (Fig. 15.4). Because each eye views an object from a different angle, the retinal images do not fall precisely on corresponding points of each retina. The disparity a three-dimensional percept to be constructed. This is termed *stereopsis*. The development of stereopsis requires that eye movements and visual alignment are coordinated over approximately the first five years of life.

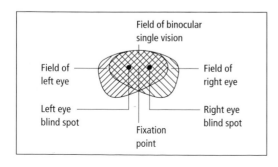

Figure 15.4 Elimination of the blind spot and increase in the field of vision that binocular single vision affords.

Binocular single vision and stereopsis afford certain advantages to the individual:
- They increase the field of vision.
- They eliminate the blind spot, since the blind spot of one eye falls in the seeing field of the other.
- They provide a binocular acuity, which is greater than monocular acuity.
- Stereopsis provides depth perception.

If the visual axes of the two eyes are not aligned, binocular single vision is not possible. This results in:
- *Diplopia*. An object is seen to be in two different places.
- *Visual confusion*. Two separate and different objects appear to be at the same point.

In children, a non-alignment of the visual axes of the two eyes (or squint) results in suppression of the image in the squinting eye. This means that when the vision in the two eyes is tested together only one object is seen and there is no diplopia. If this is prolonged and constant during the sensitive period of visual development it causes a reduced visual acuity in the squinting eye (*strabismic amblyopia*). Amblyopia will only develop if the squint constantly affects the same eye. Some children alternate the squinting eye. These children will not develop amblyopia, but they do not develop stereopsis either.

Aetiology of non-paralytic squint

Non-paralytic squint (Fig. 15.5):
1 May develop in an otherwise normal child with normal eyes. The cause of the problem in these patients remains obscure. It is thought to be caused by an abnormality in the central coordination of eye movements.
2 May be associated with ocular disease:

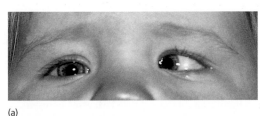

(a)

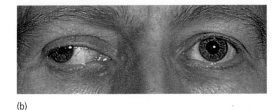

Figure 15.5 The appearance of (a) a convergent squint: right eye fixing; and (b) a divergent squint: left eye fixing. Note the position of the light reflection in each eye.

(b)

a A refractive error which prevents the formation of a clear image on the retina. This is the most common factor. If the refractive error is dissimilar in the two eyes (*anisometropia*) one retinal image will be blurred.

b Opacities in the media of the eye blurring or preventing the formation of the retinal image (i.e. corneal opacities or cataract).

c Abnormalities of the retina preventing the translation of a correctly formed image into neural impulses.

d In a child with an equal degree of long sight (hypermetropia) in both eyes a convergent squint may develop because of the *increased accommodative effort* required to focus on distant, and particularly near, objects. The link (*synkinesis*) between the accommodative and convergence mechanisms leads to an excessive convergence, and ultimately to a convergent squint of one eye. Where the squint only occurs on attempted focusing on near objects, amblyopia does not develop since binocular visual alignment remains normal for some of the time during distant viewing.

History

The presence of a squint in a child may be noted by the parents or detected at preschool or school screening clinics. It may be intermittent or constant. There may be a family history of squint or refractive error. The following should be noted:

- When the squint is present – i.e. is it constant?
- How long a squint has been present.
- Past medical, birth and family history of the child.

Examination

First the patient is observed for features that may simulate a squint. These include:
- *epicanthus* (a crescentic fold of skin on the side of the nose that incompletely covers the inner canthus);
- facial asymmetry.

Then the alignment of the two eyes is tested, using a pen torch. The corneal reflection of a torch light, held 33 cm in front of the subject, is a guide to eye position. If the child is squinting the reflection will be central in the fixating eye and deviated in the squinting eye (Fig. 15.5).

A *cover/uncover test* (Fig. 15.6) is next performed to detect a manifest squint (a *tropia*).

- The right eye is completely covered for a few seconds whilst holding a detailed near target, such as, in front of the child as a fixation target. The left eye is closely observed. If it has been maintaining fixation it should not move. If it moves

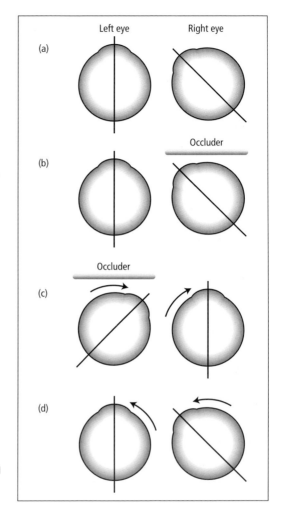

Figure 15.6 The cover/uncover test. (a) A manifest right convergent squint (right esotropia) is present. (b) The right, squinting eye, is occluded. There is no movement of the left eye, which maintains fixation. (c) The left eye is occluded. The squinting right eye moves outwards to take up fixation, and the non-squinting eye moves inwards because the movement of the two eyes is linked. (d) The cover is removed from the left eye, which moves outwards to take up fixation; the right eye moves inward to resume its squinting position. (If an alternating squint was present (i.e. each eye retained the ability to fixate) the right eye would maintain fixation and the eyes would not move when the cover was removed.)

outwards to take up fixation an *esotropia* or convergent squint is present. If it moves *inwards* to take up fixation an *exotropia* or divergent squint is present.

- The cover is removed from the right eye and then the left eye covered, this time closely observing the right. If it moves *outwards* to take up fixation an *esotropia* is present. If it moves *inwards* to take up fixation an *exotropia* is present. If there is no movement no squint is present.
- The test is repeated for a distant object sited at 6 metres and for a far-distant object. It will also reveal a vertical squint.

Investigating a squint

Summary of the steps taken in investigating a squinting child:
- Determination of acuity (see Chapter 2).
- Detection of any abnormality in eye movement.
- Detection and measurement of the squint.
- Measurement of stereopsis.
- Determination of any refractive error.
- Careful examination of the eyes, including a dilated fundus view.

If no abnormal eye movement is seen an *alternate cover test* is performed. This will reveal the presence of a latent squint (a *phoria*), which occurs only when the two eyes are not simultaneously stimulated, that is in the absence of bifoveal visual stimulation. It is not really an abnormal condition, and can be demonstrated in most people who otherwise have normal binocular single vision.
- This time the cover is moved rapidly from one eye to the other a couple of times. This dissociates the eyes (i.e. there is no longer bifoveal stimulation). The right eye is now occluded, and as the occluder is removed any movement in the *right* eye is noted. If the eye is seen to move inwards an *exophoria* (latent divergence) is present and the eye has moved inwards to take up fixation. If the eye is seen to move outwards to take up fixation an *esophoria* (latent convergence) is present. Exactly the same movements would be seen in the left eye if it were covered following dissociation.

In an eye clinic the squint can be further assessed with the synoptophore (see Chapter 2). This instrument, together with special three-dimensional pictures, can also be used to determine whether the eyes are used together and whether stereopsis is present.

Refractive error is measured following topical administration of atropine or cyclopentolate eye drops to paralyse accommodation and dilate the pupil. The eye is then examined to exclude opacities of the cornea, lens or vitreous and abnormalities of the retina or optic disc.

Treatment

A non-paralytic squint with no associated ocular disease is treated as follows:
- Any significant refractive error is first corrected with glasses.
- If amblyopia is present and the vision does not improve with glasses the better-seeing eye is patched to try and stimulate recovery of visual acuity in the amblyopic eye.
- *Surgical intervention* to realign the eyes may be required for functional reasons (to restore or establish binocular single vision) or for cosmetic reasons (to prevent a child being singled out at school) (Fig. 15.7).

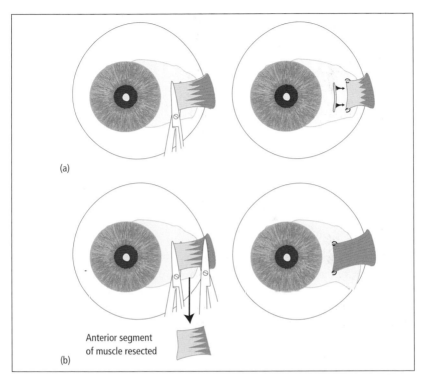

(a)

(b)

Anterior segment
of muscle resected

Figure 15.7 The principles of squint surgery. (a) Recession. The conjunctiva has been incised to expose the medial rectus muscle. The muscle is then disinserted and moved backwards on the globe. (b) Resection. Following exposure of the muscle the anterior tendon and muscle are resected, thus shortening them; the muscle is then reattached to its original position.

The principle of surgery is to realign the eyes by adjusting the position of the muscles on the globe or by shortening the muscle. Access to the muscles is gained by making a small incision in the conjunctiva.

● Moving the muscle insertion backwards on the globe (*recession*) weakens its action.
● Removing a segment of the muscle at its insertion (*resection*) strengthens its action.

Prognosis

Glasses and patching can significantly improve vision in the squinting eye. Unfortunately realignment, even if performed when the child is very young, is rarely associated with the development of stereopsis in the majority of non-paralytic squints.

The operation is important from the cosmetic viewpoint, however, particularly when the child starts school.

Paralytic squint

Isolated nerve palsy

Pathogenesis

Disease of the third, fourth and sixth nerves and their central connections gives rise to a paralytic strabismus (Fig. 15.8). Each nerve may be affected at any point along its course from brainstem nucleus to orbit. Table 15.1 details some causes.

History and examination

The patient complains of diplopia. There may be an abnormal head posture to compensate for the inability of the eye to move in a particular direction.

A third nerve palsy results in:

- failure of adduction, elevation and depression of the eye;

Table 15.1 The causes of isolated nerve palsies.

Orbital disease	e.g. neoplasia
Vascular disease	Diabetes (a 'pupil sparing' third nerve palsy, i.e. there is no mydriasis)
	Hypertension
	Aneurysm (most commonly a painful third nerve palsy from an aneurysm of the posterior communicating artery. Mydriasis is usually present)
	Caroticocavernous sinus fistula (also causes myogenic palsy)
	Cavernous sinus thrombosis
Trauma	Most common cause of fourth and sixth nerve palsy
Neoplasia	Meningioma
	Acoustic neuroma
	Glioma
Raised intracranial pressure	May cause a third or sixth nerve palsy (a false localizing sign)
Inflammation	Sarcoidosis
	Vasculitic disease (i.e. giant cell arteritis)
	Infection (particularly herpes zoster)
	Guillain–Barré syndrome

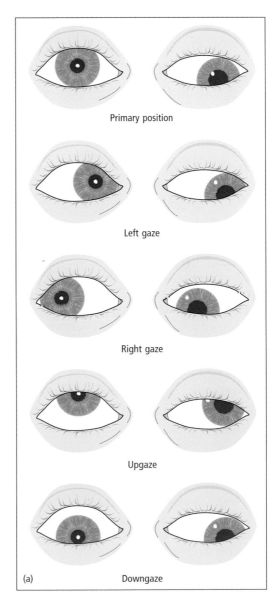

Primary position

Left gaze

Right gaze

Upgaze

(a)   Downgaze

Figure 15.8 (a) Left third nerve palsy: note the dilated pupil and ptosis as well as the limitation of eye movement.

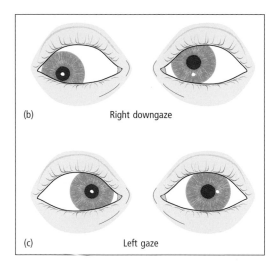

(b)   Right downgaze

(c)   Left gaze

Figure 15.8 (*continued*)
(b) Left fourth nerve palsy: the defect is maximal when the patient tries to look down when the left eye is adducted. (c) Sixth nerve palsy: the left eye is unable to abduct.

- ptosis;
- in some cases, a dilated pupil due to involvement of the autonomic fibres.

A fourth nerve palsy results in defective depression of the eye when attempted in adduction. It produces the least noticeable eye-movement abnormality. Patients may notice vertical double vision with some torsion of the image, particularly when going downstairs or reading.

A sixth nerve palsy results in failure of abduction of the eye.

Treatment

An isolated nerve palsy is often related to coexistent systemic disease. If a posterior communicating aneurysm is suspected the patient must be sent for neurosurgical review and angiography. The most common cause of a palsy is microvascular disease of a peripheral cranial nerve, itself associated with diabetes or hypertension. Here, nerve function recovers over some months and the symptoms abate.

Orbital disease (see Chapter 4) and disease in the cavernous sinus may also be the cause of multiple nerve palsies such as the third, fourth and sixth nerves, become anatomically close together. A CT or MRI scan will show the lesion (e.g. an orbital metastasis).

Diplopia can be helped by fitting prisms to the patient's glasses, which realign the retinal images. Alternatively the affected eye can be patched. If eye movements fail to improve spontaneously then surgical intervention may be required. Such intervention will seldom restore normal eye movement but is aimed at restoring an acceptable field of binocular single vision in the primary positions of gaze (i.e.

straight ahead and in downgaze), the commonest positions in which the eyes are used.

Disease of the extraocular muscles

Dysthyroid eye disease

Pathogenesis

Disorders of the thyroid gland can be associated with an infiltration of the extraocular muscles with lymphocytes and the deposition of glycosaminoglycans. An immunological process is suspected but not fully determined.

Symptoms and signs

The patient may sometimes complain of:
• A red painful eye (associated with exposure caused by proptosis). If the redness is limited to part of the eye only it may indicate active inflammation in the adjacent muscle.
• Double vision.
• Reduced visual acuity (sometimes associated with optic neuropathy).
On examination (Fig. 15.9a):
• There may be *proptosis* of the eye (the eye protrudes from the orbit, also termed *exophthalmos*).
• The eye may be *chemosed* and injected over the muscle insertions.
• The upper lid may be *retracted* so that sclera is visible (due in part to increased sympathetic activity stimulating the sympathetically innervated smooth muscle of levator). This results in a characteristic stare.
• The upper lid may lag behind the movement of the globe on downgaze (*lid lag*).

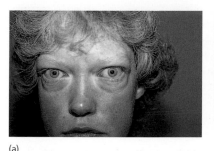
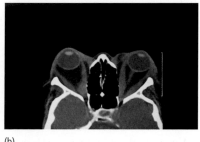

(a) (b)

Figure 15.9 Dysthyroid eye disease: (a) clinical appearance; (b) a CT scan demonstrating muscle thickening.

- There may be restricted eye movements or squint (also termed restrictive thyroid myopathy, exophthalmic ophthalmoplegia, dysthyroid eye disease or Graves' disease).

The inferior rectus is the most commonly affected muscle. Its movement becomes restricted and there is mechanical limitation of the eye in upgaze. Involvement of the medial rectus causes mechanical limitation of abduction, thereby mimicking a sixth nerve palsy. A CT or MRI scan shows enlargement of the muscles (Fig. 15.9b).

Dysthyroid eye disease is associated with two serious acute complications:

1 Excessive exposure of the conjunctiva and cornea with the formation of chemosis (oedematous swelling of the conjunctiva), and corneal ulcers due to proptosis and failure of the lids to protect the cornea. The condition may lead to corneal perforation.

2 Compressive optic neuropathy due to compression and ischaemia of the optic nerve by the thickened muscles. This leads to field loss and may cause blindness.

Treatment

Corneal exposure and optic nerve compression require urgent treatment with systemic steroids, radiotherapy or surgical orbital decompression.

In the long term, treatment may be needed for the eye-movement problems and to improve the cosmetic appearance. A period may elapse while the eye movements stabilize, during which time prisms can be used to manage the diplopia. Once stabilized, if the patient remains symptomatic, surgery on the extraocular muscles can be performed to increase the field of binocular single vision. If desired, cosmetic surgery to lower the upper lids can also be performed following the squint surgery.

Myasthenia gravis

Pathogenesis

Myasthenia gravis is caused by the development of antibodies to the acetylcholine receptors of striated muscle. It affects females more than males and although commonest in the 15–50 age group may affect young children and older adults. Some 40% of patients may show involvement of the extraocular muscles only.

Symptoms and signs

The extraocular muscles fatigue, resulting in a variable diplopia. A variable ptosis may also be present. This can be demonstrated by asking the patient to look up and down rapidly a number of times to fatigue the muscle. There may be evidence of systemic muscle weakness.

Treatment

The diagnosis can be confirmed by electromyography or by determining whether an injection of neostigmine or edrophonium (cholinesterase antagonists) temporarily restores normal muscle movement. This test must be performed under close medical supervision with resuscitation equipment and atropine to hand because of the possibility of cholinergic side effects such as bradycardia and bronchospasm.

Patients are treated, in collaboration with a neurologist, with neostigmine or pyridostigmine. Systemic steroids and surgical removal of the thymus also have a role in treatment.

Ocular myositis

This is an inflammation of the extraocular muscles associated with pain and diplopia, leading to a restriction in the movement of the involved muscle (similar to that seen in dysthyroid eye disease). It is not usually associated with systemic disease, but thyroid abnormalities should be excluded. The conjunctiva over the involved muscle is inflamed. CT or MRI scanning shows a thickening of the muscle. If symptoms are troublesome it responds to a short course of steroids.

Ocular myopathy

Ocular myopathy (progressive external ophthalmoplegia) is a rare condition where the movement of the eyes is slowly and symmetrically reduced. There is an associated ptosis. Ultimately, eye movement may be lost completely.

Brown's syndrome

The action of the superior oblique muscle may be congenitally restricted, which reduces elevation in adduction by the ipsilateral inferior oblique muscle (Brown's syndrome). The exact cause remains unknown, although it appears to involve restriction of tendon movement as it passes through the trochlear pulley. The condition may also result from trauma to the orbit.

Duane's syndrome

This is a 'congenital miswiring' of the medial and lateral rectus muscles (cases of an absent sixth nerve and nucleus are also reported). There is neuromuscular activity in the lateral rectus during adduction and reduced lateral rectus activity in abduction. This results in limited abduction and narrowing of the palpebral aperture on adduction with retraction of the eye into the globe (due to simultaneous contraction of medial and lateral rectus muscles). The condition may be unilateral or, more rarely, bilateral. Children do not usually develop amblyopia, because binocular alignment is normal in some positions of gaze, and surgical intervention is often not required.

Gaze palsies

Gage palsies affect the movement of the two eyes acting in concert. Disordered eye movement results from damage to the pathways connecting the cranial nerve nuclei together and to the higher centres. The abnormality in eye movement depends on the point at which the pathway is disrupted. Both the extent and form of eye movement may be affected. Some of the more common are briefly described below. The ophthalmologist usually investigates and manages these patients with the help of a neurologist.

Lesions of the parapontine reticular formation (PPRF)

Pathogenesis

The PPRF controls the horizontal movements of the eyes. Lesions affecting the PPRF are usually associated with other brainstem disease. It may be seen in patients with:
- vascular disease;
- tumours.

Symptoms and signs

There is:
- a failure of horizontal movements of both eyes to the side of the lesion (a *horizontal gaze palsy*);
- deviation of the eyes to the contralateral side in acute cases.

Internuclear ophthalmoplegia

Pathogenesis

It is caused by a lesion of the medial longitudinal fasciculus (MLF) (Fig. 15.10). The MLF connects the sixth nerve nucleus to the third nerve nucleus on the opposite side and coordinates their activity in gaze movements.

It may become damaged in:
- demyelination (e.g. multiple sclerosis – usually bilateral);
- vascular disease (unilateral).

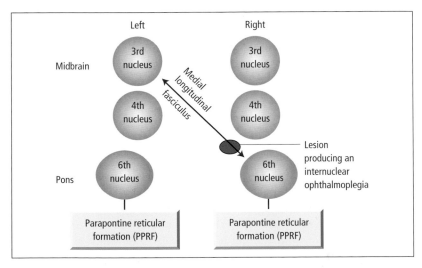

Figure 15.10 The site of the lesion producing an internuclear ophthalmoplegia.

Symptoms and signs

The patient complains of horizontal diplopia. There is a:
- reduction of adduction on the same side as the lesion;
- nystagmus of the contralateral, abducting eye.

Management

Spontaneous recovery is usual although variable in demyelination. An MRI scan may be helpful diagnostically, both to locate the causal brainstem lesion and, in demyelination, to determine whether other plaques are present.

Parinaud's syndrome (dorsal midbrain syndrome)

Pathogenesis

In Parinaud's syndrome a lesion in the dorsal midbrain involves the centre for vertical gaze. It may be seen in patients with:
- demyelination;
- space-occupying lesions such as a *pinealoma* which press on the tectum;
- infarction of the dorsal midbrain;
- an enlarged third ventricle.

Symptoms and signs

The disorder causes:
- deficient elevation of both eyes;
- convergence of the eyes and retraction into the orbit associated with nystagmus on attempted elevation;
- light–near dissociation of the pupil (the pupil constricts on accommodation but reacts poorly to a light stimulus).

Abnormal oscillations of the eyes

Nystagmus

This refers to repeated involuntary to and fro or up and down movements of the eyes. Similar movements may occur normally when following a moving object (e.g. looking out of a train window) (*optokinetic nystagmus*) or following stimulation of the vestibular system. When examined closely they may be seen to have a slow phase in one direction and a fast phase in the other (*jerk nystagmus*). The nystagmus is described as beating to the side of the fast component. In some cases the speed of eye movement may be roughly the same in either direction (*pendular nystagmus*). Jerk nystagmus may also be seen at the extreme position of gaze (*end-gaze nystagmus*).

Acquired nystagmus

Pathologically, jerk nystagmus may be seen:
- In cerebellar disease, when it is worse when gaze is directed towards the side of the lesion. The fast phase is directed towards the side of the lesion.
- With some drugs (such as barbiturates).
- In damage to the labyrinth and its central connections, when a fine jerk nystagmus results. The fast phase of the movement is away from the lesion and it is usually present only acutely.

An *upbeat* nystagmus (fast phase upwards) is commonly associated with brainstem disease. It may also be seen in toxic states, e.g. with excess alcohol intake.

A *downbeat* nystagmus may be seen in patients with a posterior fossa lesion near the cervicomedullary junction (e.g. a Chiari malformation, where cerebellar tissue is dragged through the foramen magnum). It may also be seen in patients with demyelination, and again may be present in toxic states.

Patients with nerve palsies or weakness of the extraocular muscles may develop nystagmus when looking in the direction of the affected muscle (*gaze-evoked nystagmus*). The fast phase of the movement is in the field of action of the weak muscle.

Patients with acquired nystagmus complain that the visual environment is in continual movement (*oscillopsia*).

Congenital nystagmus

Nystagmus can be congenital in origin.
- *Sensory* congenital nystagmus. Here the movements may be at similar speeds in both directions (pendular nystagmus) or of the jerk variety. It is associated with poor vision (e.g. congenital cataract, albinism).
- *Motor* congenital nystagmus is a jerk nystagmus developing at birth in children with no visual defect.

The continuous movement of the eye reduces visual acuity but does not cause oscillopsia in congenital nystagmus. The exact degree of disability depends on:
- the speed of the nystagmus;
- whether there are short periods of rest between the nystagmoid movements when objects can be focused on the fovea;
- whether the nystagmus is reduced by accommodation, as is often the case.

Some subjects find a position of the eyes which reduces the nystagmus to a minimum (the *null position*), thus maximizing visual acuity.

Key points

- In analysing eye movement problems try to determine whether there is a reduction in the range of eye movements, an abnormal position of the eyes, an abnormality in the form of eye movements, or a combination of these disorders.
- An abnormality in the range of eye movements may reflect muscular, orbital, infranuclear or supranuclear disease.
- In a child with a squint it is important to exclude intraocular pathology.
- An intracranial aneurysm may present as a painful third nerve palsy involving the pupil.

Multiple choice questions

1. Match the eye muscle to the nerve
a Lateral rectus.
b Superior rectus.
c Medial rectus.
d Inferior rectus.
e Superior oblique.
f Inferior oblique.
   i Third nerve.
   ii Fourth nerve.
   iii Sixth nerve.

2. Which of the following statements are true?

a In a non-paralytic strabismus the movement of the eyes is reduced.

b In a non-paralytic strabismus the angle of deviation is unrelated to the direction of gaze.

c In a paralytic strabismus, the eye movement is reduced.

d Nystagmus refers to an oscillating movement of the eyes.

e In a horizontal gaze palsy the patient is unable to look to one side.

3. Amblyopia

a Refers to a developmental reduction in visual acuity.

b May be caused by Duane's syndrome.

c May be caused by a previously unidentified difference in refractive correction between the two eyes.

d May be caused by a squint.

e May be treated by patching the amblyopic eye.

4. Nerve palsies affecting the third, fourth on sixth cranial nerves may be seen in

a Orbital disease.

b Raised intracranial pressure.

c Ischaemia of the cerebral cortex.

d Systemic inflammatory disease.

e Trauma.

5. Internuclear ophthalmoplegia

a Is caused by a lesion of the medial longitudinal fasciculus.

b Manifests as a reduced adduction and contralateral nystagmus in the abducting eye.

c Is manifested by a failure of the eye to elevate in adduction.

d May be caused by demyelination.

e Requires surgical treatment.

Answers

1. Match the eye muscle to the nerve

a Sixth nerve.

b Third nerve.

c Third nerve.

d Third nerve.

e Fourth nerve.

f Third nerve.

2. Which of the following statements are true?

a False. The eye movements are full but only the dominant eye is directed towards the fixation target.

b True.

c True. Paralytic strabismus is the term used if there is a problem with the extra-ocular muscles, orbital disease or a nerve palsy.

d True.

e True. Supranuclear coordination is affected. This may be seen in a patient with an acute cerebrovascular accident.

3. Amblyopia

a True.

b False. The eyes are usually aligned in some visual direction or other, so that binocular vision develops normally.

c True. If the images on the retinas are dissimilar, with one image more blurred than the other, the brain suppresses the more blurred image.

d True. If the visual axes are not aligned the brain will suppress the image from one eye.

e False. The non-amblyopic eye is patched, to improve vision in the amblyopic eye.

4. Nerve palsies affecting the third, fourth and sixth cranial nerves may be seen in

a True.

b True. The sixth cranial nerve may be compressed along its intracranial course.

c False. This will not affect the cranial nerves.

d True. It may be seen in sarcoidosis, for example.

e True. This is the most common cause of a fourth or sixth cranial nerve palsy.

5. Internuclear ophthalmoplegia

a True.

b True.

c False. This is the description of Brown's syndrome.

d True.

e False. Spontaneous resolution is usual in patients with a microvascular cause. Recovery is more variable in patients with multiple sclerosis.

Chapter 16

Trauma

Learning objectives

To be able to:
- Take a history in a case of eye trauma.

To understand:
- The effects of trauma on the eye and ocular adnexae.
- The management of penetrating eye trauma.
- The management of chemical injury to the eye.

Introduction

Although the eye is well protected by the orbit it may yet be subject to injuries (Fig. 16.1). Forms of injury include:

- Foreign bodies becoming lodged under the upper lid or on the surface of the eye, especially the cornea.
- Blunt trauma from objects small enough not to impact on the orbital rim (shuttlecocks, squash balls, champagne corks and knuckles are some of the offenders). The sudden alteration of pressure, and distortion of the eye, may cause severe damage.
- Penetrating trauma, where ocular structures are damaged by a foreign body which passes through the ocular coat and may also be retained in the eye. With the introduction of the seat belt laws the incidence of penetrating injury following road traffic accidents has declined.
- Chemical and radiation injury, where the resultant reaction of the ocular tissues causes the damage.

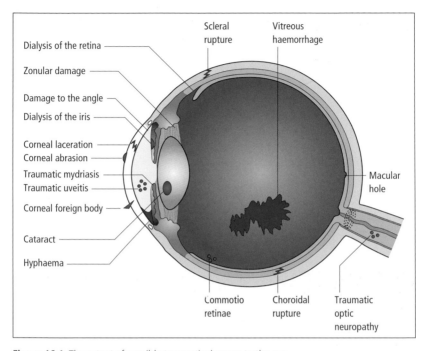

Figure 16.1 The extent of possible traumatic damage to the eye.

History, symptoms and signs

A careful history is essential.

- Use of a hammer and chisel can release a flake of metal which will penetrate the globe, leaving only a tell-tale subconjunctival haemorrhage to indicate penetration of the sclera and suggest a retained foreign body. Pain may be minor.
- A wire under tension, or a rose thorn, may penetrate the cornea briefly, sometimes creating a barely visible track.
- A blunt injury to the eye may also result in damage to the orbit (*blow-out fracture*).
- It is vitally important to determine the nature of any chemical that may have been in contact with the eye. Strong alkalis penetrate the anterior tissues of the eye and may rapidly cause irreversible damage.

The patient's symptoms will relate to the degree and type of trauma suffered. Pain, lacrimation and blurring of vision are common features of trauma, but mild symptoms may disguise a potentially blinding intraocular foreign body. As in all history taking, it is essential to enquire about previous ocular and medical history.

Examination

Without a slit lamp

The examination will depend on the type of injury. In all cases it is important that visual acuity is recorded in the injured and *uninjured* eye for medico-legal reasons among others. Where a penetrating injury is suspected and pressure to the globe must be avoided, it may only be possible to measure vision approximately in the injured eye; the patient may be able to detect light shone through the closed lid. The skin around the orbit and eyelids should be carefully examined for a penetrating wound.

Orbital injury

Damage to the orbit itself (a *blow-out fracture*; Fig. 16.2) is suspected if the following signs are present:

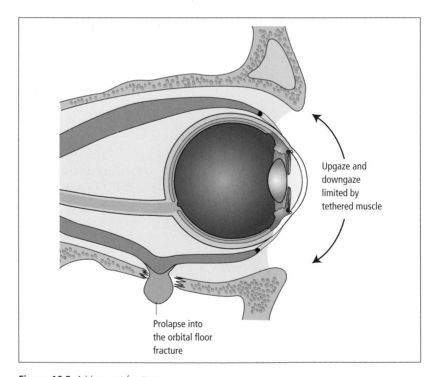

Upgaze and downgaze limited by tethered muscle

Prolapse into the orbital floor fracture

Figure 16.2 A blow-out fracture.

Symptoms and signs of a penetrating eye injury

- History of high-velocity object hitting the eye.
- Dark tissue in the cornea or sclera (iris plugging of a penetrating wound).
- Distortion of the pupil.
- Unusually deep anterior chamber.
- Cataract.
- Vitreous haemorrhage.

- Emphysema (air in the skin which crackles when pressed) derived from a fractured sinus.
- A patch of paraesthesia below the orbital rim suggesting infraorbital nerve damage. The infraorbital nerve is commonly injured in orbital blow-out injury involving the floor of the orbit.
- Limitation of eye movements, particularly on upgaze and downgaze, due to trapping of the inferior rectus muscle by connective-tissue septa caught in the fractured site (in the inferior orbital floor, the most commonly fractured).
- Subsequently the eye may become recessed into the orbit (*enophthalmos*).
- If the lid margin is cut at the medial canthus it is important to determine if either of the lacrimal canaliculi is severed, causing epiphora if untreated.

Further examination of a traumatized eye will require the instillation of a local anaesthetic to facilitate lid opening (lignocaine, amethocaine). If a penetrating eye injury is suspected it is important that no pressure is applied to the globe, to avoid expression of its contents.

The conjunctiva and sclera

These must be examined for the presence of any lacerations. If the history is appropriate a subconjunctival haemorrhage should be considered to be the potential site of a scleral perforation (Fig. 16.3). The fundus should be examined with full mydriasis.

If a chemical injury has occurred the conjunctiva may appear white and ischaemic (Fig. 16.4). If such changes are extensive, involving the greater part of the limbal circumference, corneal healing will be grossly impaired because of damage to the epithelial stem cells and there will be additional complications such as uveitis, secondary glaucoma and cataract.

The cornea

This is examined for loss of the epithelial layer (abrasion), for lacerations and for foreign bodies (Fig. 16.5). The instillation of fluorescein will identify the extent of

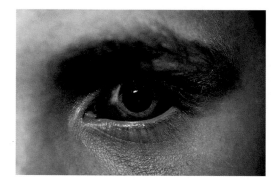

Figure 16.3 A subconjunctival haemorrhage.

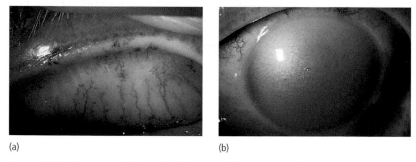

(a)   (b)

Figure 16.4 (a) An everted lid showing ischaemia of the upper tarsal conjunctiva following an alkali burn; (b) a hazy cornea following an alkali burn.

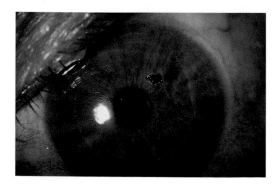

Figure 16.5 A corneal foreign body. (With permission from Sue Ford, Western Eye Hospital.)

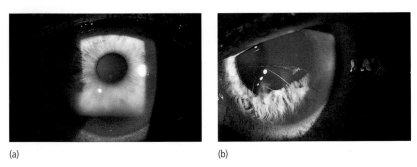

(a)   (b)

Figure 16.6 (a) A hyphaema; (b) penetrating eye injury (note the eyelashes in the anterior chamber and the distorted iris).

an abrasion and, if concentrated, will identify a leak of aqueous through a penetrating wound (see Chapter 2). If the globe appears intact and a subtarsal foreign body is suspected (signalled by fine, vertical, linear corneal abrasions) the upper lid must be everted (see Fig. 2.7). This exposes the underside of the lid and allows any foreign body to be identified and removed.

Electromagnetic radiation may injure the conjunctiva and the cornea. Unprotected exposure to ultraviolet radiation from an arc lamp (*arc eye*) or sunlamp, or reflected from snow, is the commonest cause of this severely painful condition. Typically, ocular pain onsets acutely, six hours after exposure to the radiation, and the cornea shows diffuse epithelial oedema and punctate damage which resolves within 24–48 hours.

The anterior chamber

Blunt trauma may cause haemorrhage into the anterior chamber, where it collects with a fluid level becoming visible (*hyphaema*). This is caused by rupture of the root of the iris blood vessels, or the iris may be torn away from its insertion into the ciliary body (*iris dialysis*) to produce a D-shaped pupil. Hyphaema may also be seen with a penetrating eye injury, and the shape of the pupil may be distorted if the peripheral iris has plugged a penetrating corneal wound (Fig. 16.6). The pupil may also show a fixed dilatation as a result of blunt trauma (*traumatic mydriasis*).

The lens

Dislocation of the lens following blunt trauma may be suggested by a fluttering of the iris diaphragm on eye movement (*iridodonesis*). Lens clarity should be assessed with the slit lamp and against the red reflex after pupil dilation. Cataracts develop abruptly with direct penetrating trauma (Fig. 16.7). Blunt trauma also causes a posterior subcapsular cataract within hours of injury, which may be transient.

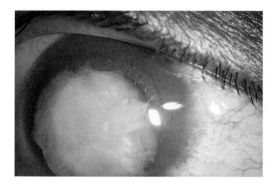

Figure 16.7 The lens in this patient has become disrupted and cataractous following penetrating trauma.

The fundus

The fundus should be inspected with a direct ophthalmoscope after full mydriasis. If no neurological complications accompany the injury and ocular penetration is not suspected, the pupil can be dilated. Areas of retinal haemorrhage and whiteness (oedema) may be seen (*commotio retinae*). A *retinal dialysis* (a separation of the peripheral retina from its junction with the pars plana of the ciliary body) and a macular hole (see Chapter 11) may also result from blunt trauma. The choroid may also become torn; acutely, this may cause sub-retinal haemorrhage which is then followed by the development of sub-retinal scarring. Peripheral retinal changes can only be excluded with indirect ophthalmoscopy or slit-lamp microscopy. If there is no red reflex and no fundus details are visible, this suggests a vitreous haemorrhage.

The optic disc may be pale from a traumatic optic neuropathy caused by avulsion of the blood vessels supplying the optic nerve. Although this is uncommon, it leads to a profound loss of vision. No treatment is available.

With a slit lamp

The slit lamp allows a more detailed examination to be performed, which may reveal:
- A shallow anterior chamber compared to the fellow eye, suggesting an anterior penetrating injury with aqueous loss.
- A microscopic hyphaema, where red cells are present, circulating in the anterior chamber, but have not settled to form a hyphaema level.
- The presence of white cells in the anterior chamber (*traumatic uveitis*).
- *Recession* of the iridocorneal angle seen with a gonioscopic contact lens (the ciliary muscle apex is disinserted from the scleral spur and moves posteriorly). This may be seen with blunt trauma and result in raised intraocular pressure.

• Raised intraocular pressure measured by applanation tonometry. This may accompany a hyphaema or lens dislocation.

Treatment

Lacerations to the skin and lids

These require careful suturing, particularly if the lid margin is involved. If one of the lacrimal canaliculi is damaged an attempt can be made to repair it, but if repair is unsuccessful usually the remaining tear duct is capable of draining all the tears. If both canaliculi are involved, an attempt at repair should always be made.

Corneal abrasions

This is an extremely painful condition which normally heals rapidly. It should be treated with antibiotic ointment, with or without an eye pad. Dilation of the pupil with cyclopentolate 1% can help to relieve the pain caused by spasm of the ciliary muscle.

Recurrent corneal abrasions when such an injury, is caused by flexible objects such as fingernails, twigs or the edge of a newspaper, a minority of patients may be troubled by recurrent episodes of pain, particularly in the early hours of the morning or on waking. This condition is termed *recurrent corneal erosion* and is due to a defective adhesion of the resurfacing epithelium to Bowman's layer at the site of injury. Prophylaxis against further recurrent corneal erosions is attempted by using a lubricating ointment at night for several weeks after an initial attack, but more permanent results are achieved by inducing a subepithelial scar at the site of the original injury to bind the sub-epithelial layer to Bowmans layer. This can be induced by laser treatment or by applying a series of micropunctures with a needlepoint to the affected zone.

UV injury to the cornea responds quickly to topical steroids.

Corneal foreign bodies

Corneal foreign bodies should be removed with a needle under topical anaesthesia (Fig. 16.8); a rust ring may remain and can be removed with a small, rotating burr. Subtarsal objects can often be swept away with a cotton-wool bud from the everted lid. The patient is then treated as for an abrasion. If there is any suggestion that a foreign body may have penetrated the globe the eye must be carefully examined with dilation of the pupil to allow a good view of the lens and retina. An X-ray with the eyes looking up and then down, or a CT scan, may also be indicated if an intraocular foreign body is suspected. Microsurgical techniques can be used to remove foreign bodies from the eye under direct view.

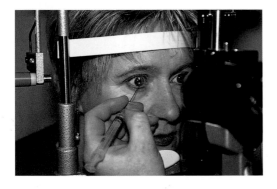

Figure 16.8 Removal of a superficial ocular foreign body at the slit lamp.

Corneal and scleral penetrating trauma

Once identified, no further examination of the globe should be performed but a shield should be gently placed over the eye and the patient referred for urgent ophthalmic treatment. These serious injuries, often with grave implications for sight, require careful microsurgical suturing to restore the integrity of the globe. Once the eye has settled from this primary repair additional operations are often required, to:

- remove a cataract;
- remove a foreign body;
- repair a detached retina or remove the vitreous gel to prevent this occurrence.

Occasionally, in the longer term, the fellow eye may develop sympathetic ophthalmitis (see Chapter 9).

Uveitis

This responds to the usual treatment with steroids and dilating drops. It may be accompanied by elevated intraocular pressure requiring additional medical treatment.

Hyphaema

This usually settles with rest, but a rebleed may occur in the first 5–6 days after injury. Children usually require admission to hospital for a few days, while adults can be treated at home provided they can rest and no complications develop. Steroid eye drops are given for a short time, together with dilation of the pupil. Steroids reduce the risk of rebleeds. The commonest complication is a raised ocular pressure, particularly if there is a secondary bleed, which tends to be more severe than the first. It is for this reason that rest is important. Raised pressure usually responds to medical treatment, but occasionally surgical intervention is required. When the hyphaema has settled it is important that the eye is carefully checked for other complications of blunt trauma. Hyphaema clears more slowly after trauma in patients with sickle cell disease because the hypoxic and acidic environment within the anterior chamber precipitates sickling, and sickling retards red cell removal via the trabecular meshwork.

Retinal damage

In *commotio retinae* the affected zone of retina opacifies and obscures the underlying choroidal detail. It usually resolves, but requires careful observation since retinal holes may develop in affected areas and may lead to subsequent retinal detachment.

Retinal dialysis requires surgical intervention to repair any detached retina.

A *vitreous haemorrhage* may absorb over several weeks, or may require removal by vitrectomy. An ultrasound scan is useful in detecting associated retinal detachments.

Chemical injury

The most important part of the treatment is to irrigate the eye immediately with copious quantities of clean water at the time of the accident. This must be repeated when ophthalmic care is available, when it is also important to irrigate under the upper and lower lid to remove solid particles, e.g. lime. The nature of the chemical can then be ascertained by history and measuring tear pH with litmus paper. Administration of steroid and dilating drops may be required. Vitamin C, given both orally and topically, may improve healing. Systemic and topical anticollagenases may be needed (e.g. tetracyclines).

Extensive damage to the limbus may prevent resurfacing of the cornea with epithelium. A prolonged epithelial defect may lead to a corneal 'melt' (keratolysis). This is treated by limbal transplantation (which provides a new source of stem cells) or an overlay with amniotic membrane (which expands the remaining stem cells).

Orbital blow-out fracture

If a blow-out fracture is suspected, a CT scan will delineate the bony and soft-tissue injury. If this is not possible then plain orbital X-rays are performed. Treatment may be delayed until the periorbital swelling has settled. At this later stage the degree of enophthalmos and the limitation of eye movement can be measured. If the enophthalmos is cosmetically unacceptable or eye movements are significantly limited, then surgical repair of the orbital fracture is indicated.

Although some surgeons advocate an early intervention to obtain the best results, many patients will require no surgery at all.

Prognosis

The eye heals well following minor trauma and there are rarely long-term sequelae save for the occurrence of the *recurrent corneal erosion* syndrome. Penetrating ocular trauma, however, is often associated with severe visual damage and may require extensive surgery. Long-term retention of iron foreign bodies may destroy retinal function by the generation of free radicals. Similarly, chemical injuries to the eyes can result in severe long-term visual impairment and ocular discomfort. Blunt trauma can cause untreatable visual loss if a retinal hole develops at the fovea. Vision will also be impaired if the choroid at the macula is damaged. In the longer term, secondary glaucoma can develop in an eye several years after the initial insult if the trabecular meshwork has been damaged. Severe orbital trauma may also cause both cosmetic and oculomotor problems.

Key points

- Take an accurate history.
- Foreign bodies can often be found under the upper lid.
- Persistent pain in an intact eye suggests a subtarsal foreign body.
- Irrigate chemical injuries immediately with clean water.
- Suspect a perforating eye injury if the pupil is not round, a cataract has developed rapidly or a vitreous haemorrhage is present.

Multiple choice questions

1. Orbital injury may produce the following signs
a Periorbital emphysema.
b Limitation of eye movements.
c Exophthalmos in the longer term.
d A patch of anaesthesia below the orbital rim.
e Hyphaema.

2. A subconjunctival haemorrhage
a Is never associated with serious eye disease.
b May cause blood to pass into the cornea.
c Is usually associated with a reduced vision.

d May be associated with some discomfort of the eye.
e Usually settles in a couple of weeks.

3. Chemical eye injuries

a Acids cause more severe damage than alkalis.
b Initial treatment requires copious irrigation of the eye with litres of water.
c May be associated with a melt of the cornea.
d A white eye is a sign that the eye has not been severely affected.
e May be treated with oral and topical vitamin C and tetracyclines.

4. A hyphaema

a Is a fluid collection of white cells in the anterior chamber.
b May be associated with a low intraocular pressure.
c Is treated with restriction of activity.
d If it recurs within a short time may result in more severe problems.
e Is treated with steroid drops.

Answers

1. Orbital injury may produce the following signs

a True.
b True. There may be swelling of the orbital contents, or the muscle or orbital tissue may become tethered in the orbital fracture.
c False. The eye is usually recessed into the orbit (enophthalmos).
d True. This occurs with an orbital blow-out affecting the floor of the orbit, which damages the infraorbital nerve.
e True. It is always important to look at the eye closely in patients with an orbital fracture.

2. A subconjunctival haemorrhage

a False. In traumatic disease it may overlie a penetrating wound.
b False.
c False. If vision is reduced another cause must be found.
d True. It may cause slight elevation of the conjunctiva.
e True.

3. Chemical eye injuries

a False. Alkalis diffuse more rapidly and so cause the worst injuries.
b True. The area under the eyelids must also be inspected and irrigated.
c True.

d False. This may indicate a severe ischaemic injury by an alkali.
e True.

4. A hyphaema

a False. This is a hypopyon. A hyphaema is a collection of red cells.
b False. It may be associated with a raised intraocular pressure, due to an obstruction of the trabecular meshwork.
c True.
d True. A rebleed is often worse.
e True.

Chapter 17

Tropical ophthalmology: eye diseases in the developing world

Learning objectives

To understand:
- The severity of the problems associated with ophthalmic disease in developing countries.
- How these problems are being addressed.
- The clinical presentation and treatment of the major diseases, including trachoma, onchocerciasis and xerophthalmia.

Introduction

In the year 2000, 45 million of the world population were estimated to be blind, with a visual acuity of less than 3/60 or a visual field less than 10 degrees from the centre of fixation. Sixty per cent had treatable cataract or refractive error and 15% had preventable diseases such as trachoma, onchocerciasis and vitamin A deficiency. A further 25% had diabetic eye disease, glaucoma and age-related macular degeneration. Thus, while this figure grows by some 1 to 2 million each year, 75% of world blindness is treatable or preventable. Ninety per cent of the blind live in the poorest parts of the developing world.

Reasons for differences in the severity of ophthalmic disease in developed and developing countries

- Scope of disease differs.
- Prevention (for example measles immunization) programmes are usually not advanced.
- Facilities and trained personnel are often absent.

Causes of childhood blindness

- Vitamin A deficiency.
- Trachoma.
- Congenital cataract.
- Ophthalmia neonatorum.
- Congenital glaucoma.
- Congenital malformations.
- Measles.
- Retinopathy of prematurity.
- Other infections (cornea and ocular, e.g. toxoplasmosis).

There are estimated to be 1.5 million blind children in the world. Half a million children become blind each year. In developing countries where vitamin A deficiency is prevalent 50% die within two years of becoming blind. Half of all blindness in children is avoidable or treatable.

To combat worldwide blindness, in 1999 the International Agency for the Prevention of Blindness and the World Health Organization launched *Vision 2020 – the Right to Sight*. The aim of the programme is to eliminate world blindness by 2020. Many of the diseases responsible for world blindness have been discussed earlier in this book. This chapter focuses on those tropical diseases that are the major causes of preventable blindness, and on some of the methods for delivering care in the developing world.

Providing eye care in the developing world

With so much treatable and preventable eye disease, the greatest problems surrounding eye care in the developing world are:
- Dealing with environmental factors that predispose to disease.
- The cost of providing care.
- Delivering eye care to remote and widely spread populations.
- Delivering a high-quality service that is assessed and constantly improved.
- Sustaining the programme.

Cataract

Cataract is the commonest cause of treatable blindness, responsible for 17 million blind people worldwide (Fig. 17.1). The surgical methods available have been described in Chapter 8. In the developing world extracapsular cataract extraction remains the surgery of choice, as it is cheaper than phacoemulsification and less dependent on high-tech equipment. The results of surgery are excellent, and the

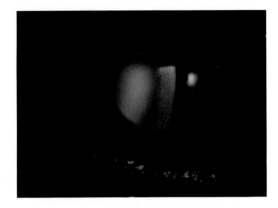

Figure 17.1 The appearance of a cataract.

challenge is to make it available. The cost of the operation, and availability of trained staff, particularly in rural communities, are major problems that have to be overcome. Various models have been developed.

In India, where cataract blindness remains a significant problem, the Aravind Eye Care system has created a highly efficient, high-volume, low-cost, self-financing system for performing cataract surgery. The system uses income from the relatively rich to pay for the very poor, who receive free surgery. Patients are screened in eye camps, and those in need of surgery or other treatment are referred to hospital.

At the Kikuyu Hospital in Kenya cataract operations are performed both by ophthalmologists and by technicians trained in surgery. The hospital also has a training programme, which is vital if the service is to be sustainable. Again, outreach clinics are used to screen patients, and those requiring surgery are transported to hospital. Seventy-five per cent of the cost of this service comes from fees; donations have helped develop the service.

As with all health programmes, it is important first to understand the epidemiology of the problem so that appropriate resources can be determined. There has been increasing emphasis on training local healthcare workers to run programmes, with outside aid providing equipment, consumables and training rather than direct surgical input. Additionally, assessment of the outcome of surgery is emphasized, to maximize the quality of care provided and match that in the developed world.

Tropical diseases

Trachoma

This is caused by *Chlamydia trachomatis*. The disease was first described in Egypt in the sixteenth century. It has not been seen in Europe since the early twentieth

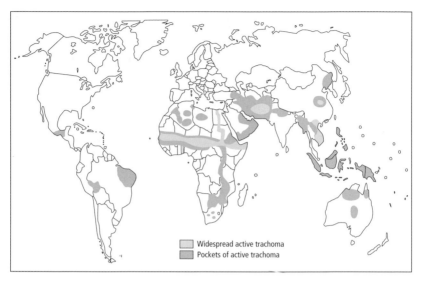

Figure 17.2 The worldwide distribution of trachoma.

century but was present in America until the 1960s. It affects more than 84 million people worldwide, mostly in dry hot parts of the developing world (Fig. 17.2) and is responsible for 3% of world blindness. In some developing communities some 60% of children are affected by active disease. It is endemic in areas of water shortage, where living conditions are crowded and hygiene poor. Flies and hand-to-eye contact spread the organisms from infected eyes. A single infection does not cause serious disease. Initially follicles (collections of lymphocytes) are present on the superior tarsus (Fig. 17.3). Papillae then appear, and the cornea is invaded by superficial vessels (pannus) with the development of peripheral scarring (Fig. 17.4). Secondary infections occur, which, together with lid deformity and trichiasis, make the corneal changes significantly worse. Continued re-infection leads to chronic corneal scarring and blindness. This results from:

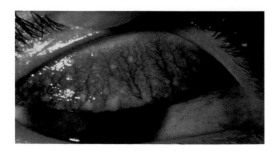

Figure 17.3 Follicles on the upper tarsus of a patient with trachoma.

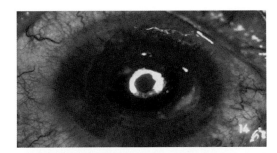

Figure 17.4 Peripheral corneal scarring in trachoma.

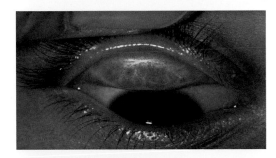

Figure 17.5 Scarring of the tarsal conjunctiva in trachoma.

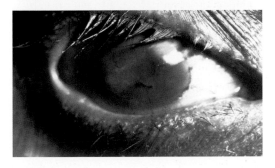

Figure 17.6 Upper lid entropion and corneal scarring in trachoma.

- Dry eye. Conjunctival scarring (Fig. 17.5) blocks lacrimal and meibomian gland duct orifices, leading to tear reduction and excessive evaporative loss.
- Reduced lubrication through loss of goblet cell mucin.
- Corneal trauma, due to cicatricial entropion (the lid margins are turned in by tarsal scarring; Fig. 17.6). This also predisposes to secondary bacterial and fungal corneal infection and scarring.

Treatment relies on:
- Public-health intervention.
- Antibiotic therapy.
- Surgery.
- A clean environment to reduce the fly population.

245

● Frequent face washing reduces transmission of the disease: the flies are less likely to be attracted to the child, and the child is less likely to spread *Chlamydia* by direct contact.

A single dose of oral azithromycin is effective in treating infected individuals, but the disease must be eradicated from all individuals in a community to prevent re-infection, and treatment must be repeated yearly. This is expensive, and the disease will recur unless changes are made to the environment in which the organism prospers. These are much harder to achieve.

In those with entropion caused by chronic disease, lid surgery is effective in everting the lid.

Onchocerciasis (river blindness)

Onchocerca volvulus, a filarial nematode, is responsible for this disease, which is found principally in Africa and South America (Fig. 17.7). Some two million people are thought to be visually impaired by the disease. Microfilariae in the skin are ingested when the female blackfly (*Simulium* sp., e.g. *S. damnosum*) bites a human for a blood meal. The microfilariae develop into infective larvae in the fly, pass to its mouth, and are then transmitted to a human with the next bite. Following moulting, the larvae develop into adult worms. Adult worms are found in subcutaneous skin nodules (onchocercomata), and diagnosis may be made from skin-snip biopsies. Alternatively, antibodies may be detected in the blood, and PCR

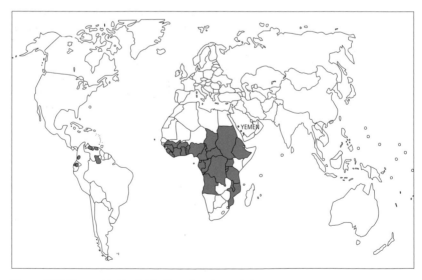

Figure 17.7 The worldwide distribution of onchocerciasis.

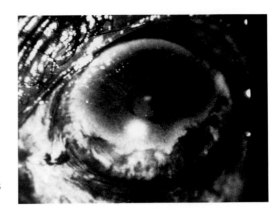

Figure 17.8 Sclerosing keratitis in onchocerciasis.

techniques have also been used to detect filarial DNA in skin scrapings. The adult worm living in the human has a lifespan of 9–14 years; the female is 30–80 cm long and the male 3–5 cm long. A female worm may produce 1600 microfilariae a day and generate a body load of 150 million. These migrate in the dermis and its lymphatics. They die after a couple of years if they do not pass into a blackfly.

It is the microfilariae that are responsible for ocular disease, entering the eye directly from the conjunctiva or from the bloodstream. The living organisms inhibit the host's immune response to them. Microfilariae are visible in the cornea, anterior chamber, vitreous and retina. Living, mobile microfilariae may be seen in the anterior chamber on biomicroscopy. In the cornea a characteristic fluffy, punctate stromal keratitis occurs as an early sign of eye disease, each opacity representing the reaction around a dead microfilarium. With increased load this advances to complete opacification (sclerosing keratitis) and consequent blindness (Fig. 17.8). Uveitis may be associated with anterior and posterior synechiae (Fig. 17.9), cataract and secondary glaucoma. Involvement of the retina and choroid are common causes of blindness (Fig. 17.10), as is optic neuritis, leading to optic atrophy.

Treatment relies on:
- Public-health intervention.
- Antibiotic therapy.

Water courses provide the breeding ground for the blackfly, which is why those whose work or daily life takes them to the banks of rivers are most at risk of infection. Control programmes are aimed at the blackfly vector, spraying its habitat with larvicides. The onchocerciasis control programme has been successful in the West African region. A low density of human population (principally farming and fishing communities) in affected areas increases the likelihood of multiple blackfly bites. Protective clothing reduces the possibility of bites but may not always be practical. Vector control programmes are a long-term proposition because the

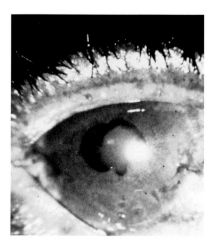

Figure 17.9 Uveitis with synechiae formed between iris and lens in onchocerciasis.

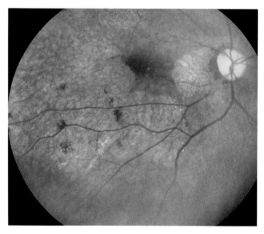

Figure 17.10 The appearance of retinal disease in onchocerciasis.

female worm lives for 9–14 years, producing ongoing microfilarial infiltration of the skin.

Ivermectin is a filaricide which has revolutionized the treatment of onchocerciasis. It is safe and effective in killing microfilariae, and reactions, if they occur, are mild and diminish with repeated dosing. It also reduces the number of adult worms present and their reproductive capability. It is given once a year, often on a community basis. Reduction in the number of microfilariae reduces the infectious potential of the blackfly and complements vector control programmes. Over 24 million people are treated each year as a result of a donation of the drug by the manufacturer, Merck, and collaborations with national and international health organizations.

Vitamin A deficiency (xerophthalmia)

Vitamin A is an essential vitamin, required for cell maturation and division and the maintenance and protection of mucosal surfaces. Dietary carotenoids from dark, leafy green vegetables, carrots, red palm oil, mangos and papayas etc. are broken down to release vitamin A (roughly 12 molecules of β-carotene for every molecule of vitamin A). Pre-formed vitamin A is available in breast milk, liver, fish oils, eggs and dairy products. Vitamin A is stored chiefly in the liver. Animal sources of the vitamin are often not available in the developing world, and environmental factors are crucial to a good diet. Social factors are also important, since poor water supply may lead to chronic diarrhoea and malabsorption, which exacerbates any deficiency. Lack of vitamin A increases susceptibility to these diseases. Deficiency in vitamin A, when associated with protein malnutrition and febrile illnesses such as measles, gives rise to severe disease.

Vitamin A deficiency causes blinding ocular disease (xerophthalmia) and an increased morbidity and mortality, particularly in preschool children over the age of 1 year, but also in pregnant women, whose nutritional requirement is increased during gestation and breastfeeding. About 140 million children suffer from vitamin A deficiency and some 5–10 million develop xerophthalmia each year, with loss of sight in half a million. The peak incidence occurs between 3 and 5 years of age. There is a widespread distribution of clinical and subclinical disease, with much of the clinical disease seen in Africa (Fig. 17.11).

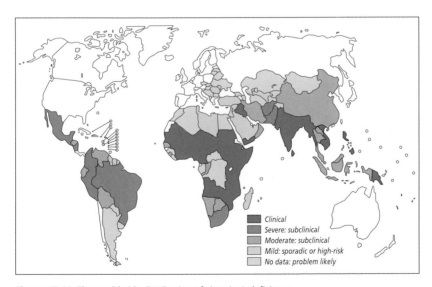

Figure 17.11 The worldwide distribution of vitamin A deficiency.

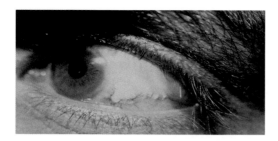

Figure 17.12 The appearance of a Bitot's spot.

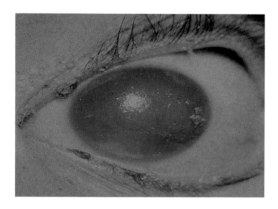

Figure 17.13 Xerosis of the cornea in vitamin A deficiency.

The features of xerophthalmia occur in the following sequence with increasing vitamin A deficiency:

• Night blindness: often the earliest symptom.

• Conjunctival xerosis: keratinization, thickening and non-wetting of the conjunctiva, frequently with Bitot's spots (Fig. 17.12) (foamy triangular surface plaques containing keratinized cells and saprophytic bacteria).

• Corneal xerosis: punctate or diffuse drying of the cornea (Fig. 17.13), usually with stromal oedema, which may progress to:

• Corneal ulceration or focal melting (keratomalacia; Fig. 17.14). This occurs in more severe disease, leading to perforation, loss of the eye and *phthisis bulbi*.

Night blindness, conjunctival and corneal xerosis are usually completely reversed by vitamin A therapy, and even corneal ulceration may be checked, leaving residual scarring.

Treatment with vitamin A supplementation, fortification of food or increasing the natural dietary intake is very cost-effective. A protein-rich diet is also advised, if possible. Delivery of supplements is often combined with immunization programmes. Education about breastfeeding, diet and food preparation is also

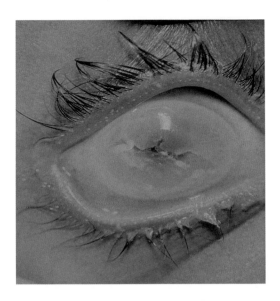

Figure 17.14 Severe corneal disease with ulceration in vitamin A deficiency.

important. Care should be taken in women of childbearing age, as vitamin A in large doses may have teratogenic effects. For this reason, maternal supplements are recommended in the immediate postpartum period, when they may replenish maternal liver stores and ensure a supply of the vitamin in the breast milk.

Measles

This is an important cause of corneal scarring and childhood blindness, and its severity is exacerbated by vitamin A deficiency. During infection with measles vitamin A stores are significantly depleted, which can result in severe corneal disease (Fig. 17.15). Vitamin A deficiency also increases the mortality from this disease. Associated exposure keratopathy, herpes simplex keratitis and other secondary infections may also cause corneal opacification, which may be compounded by

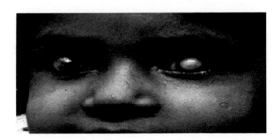

Figure 17.15 Bilateral severe corneal scarring in measles.

treatment with local remedies which traumatize the eye, or cause infection or chemical burns.

Immunization programmes will help to reduce blindness from measles.

Corneal ulceration

With so many involved in agricultural labour in the developing world, microbial keratitis, initiated by minor eye trauma, is not unusual. In northern climates, where agricultural injuries are less frequent, fungal infections are rare. But in tropical zones fungal keratitis may account for over 80% of infected cases. It is estimated that 1.5 million new cases of unilateral visual impairment due to corneal ulceration occur each year. Treatment can be expensive and is often delayed in the developing world; some topical anti-fungal agents are highly toxic and may leave their own sequelae; corneal grafting for central scarring is seldom available. Antibiotic treatment of minor eye trauma has, however, an important role in preventing progression to a bacterial keratitis.

HIV and AIDS

Treatment available in the developed world, which has reduced the severity of ocular disease associated with opportunistic infection such as CMV (see Chapter 9), is becoming available to much of the developing world. Other systemic manifestations of the disease may however occur before the CD4+ T-lymphocyte count is sufficiently low for ocular disease to become apparent.

Ophthalmia neonatorum

Infection of a child's eye occurring during birth may lead to blindness within the first month of life (see Chapter 7). The infant presents with conjunctivitis and discharge. Although a number of bacteria may be responsible for infection the two most important are:
- *Neisseria gonorrhoeae.*
- *Chlamydia trachomatis.*

Gonorrhoeal keratitis may rapidly progress to corneal perforation and endophthalmitis. Chlamydial infection is the commonest cause and the associated keratitis, if untreated, may progress to corneal scarring. It can also be associated with a pneumonitis. Because of the systemic implications of these eye infections, both are treated with systemic and topical antibiotics.

Topical prophylaxis with povidone–iodine eye drops is a simple and cost-effective means of preventing either disease.

Key points

- There were 45 million blind people in the world in the year 2000.
- Seventy-five per cent of this blindness is preventable or treatable.
- Ninety per cent of the world's blind population live in the poorest parts of the developing world.
- Vision 2020 is a worldwide programme set up to eliminate world blindness.
- Preventable forms of treatable blindness include cataract, trachoma, onchocerciasis and vitamin A deficiency.
- Treatment relies as much on education and environmental changes as on drug therapy.

Multiple choice questions

1. In the developing world
a 60% of blindness is treatable.
b 10% of blindness is treatable.
c 15% is preventable.
d 30% is preventable.

2. Trachoma
a Affects more than 84 million people.
b In some developing communities 60% of children have active disease.
c Corneal scarring may result from cicatricial entropion.
d Is treated with ivermectin.
e Follicles are present on the upper tarsus in early disease.

3. Onchocerciasis
a Is caused by a bacterium.
b Causes visual impairment in 2 million people.
c Is transmitted by the blackfly.
d Does not affect the cornea.
e Eye disease is caused by microfilariae.

4. Vitamin A deficiency (xerophthalmia)
a Affects 140 million children.
b The peak incidence for xerophthalmia is at age 10–15 years.
c Does not affect night vision.
d Bitot's spots are a specific sign.
e The severity of the disease is increased with concurrent measles infection.

Answers

1. In the developing world
a True.
b False.
c True.
d False.

2. Trachoma
a True.
b True.
c True.
d False. Trachoma is treated with a single dose of azithromycin. This needs to be repeated yearly to prevent re-infection.
e True.

3. Onchocerciasis
a False. Onchocerciasis is caused by a filarial nematode.
b True.
c True.
d False. It may result in a sclerosing keratitis with complete opacification of the cornea.
e True.

4. Vitamin A deficiency (xerophthalmia)
a True.
b False. The peak incidence is at 3–5 years.
c False. This is an early sign of the disease.
d True.
e True.

Chapter 18

The symptoms of eye disease

Learning objectives

To be able to formulate differential diagnoses for the presenting symptoms of a red eye, sudden and acute loss of vision, ocular pain and diplopia.

Introduction

So far we have looked at eye disease anatomically. This is not, however, how patients present. In this chapter, therefore, we examine presenting symptoms and how to formulate a differential diagnosis from the history.

The common symptoms of red eye, sudden or chronic visual disturbance, ocular pain and diplopia will be explored. It is important in ophthalmology, as in all medical specialties, to take a full history and note symptoms in other systems. Past medical history, drug history and family history may all yield important information and should not be overlooked (Table 18.1).

Red eye

A red eye is one of the most common presenting complaints in ophthalmology. It means redness of the exposed white of the eye, i.e. the exposed conjunctiva and underlying sclera. It is associated with infection, inflammation, trauma and acute elevation of intraocular pressure (Table 18.2).

Determining associated symptoms will help establish the diagnosis (Table 18.3).

Table 18.1 Key points in the ophthalmic history.

Consider the symptoms carefully
How long have they been present?
Are they continuous or intermittent?
What precipitated them?
What makes them better or worse?
How are they changing?
Are there associated symptoms?
Is there a history of previous eye, or relevant systemic disease?
Is there a relevant drug history, family history or social history? (alcohol, smoking, exposure to chemicals)

Table 18.2 Red eye: causes and symptoms.

Major causes	Trauma
	Infection
	Acute glaucoma
	Other forms of inflammation
Associated symptoms	Discharge
	Pain
	Photophobia
	Blurred vision

Trauma

A traumatic cause is usually obvious. Your history should note details of the trauma and whether this was due to blunt injury, a sharp object or a high-speed projectile. High-speed metal fragments from hammering may penetrate the globe and threaten sight.

• *Subconjunctival haemorrhage* is bright red due to exposure to ambient oxygen levels, and obscures the white of the sclera. It may be traumatic or spontaneous, or may be associated with systemic hypertension or blood clotting disorders including anticoagulant therapy (the INR may need checking).

• *Corneal foreign bodies* and *abrasions* cause extreme pain and epiphora. Sensory innervation is nociceptive, and higher than in any other part of the body, e.g. it is 400 times greater than in the fingertip. Corneal injury stimulates reflex antidromic vasodilatation of limbal episcleral vessels, termed a *limbal* or *ciliary* flush. This characteristic sign is often in the meridian of the lesion, aiding its detection, or it may surround the limbus when trauma is associated with iritis. Trauma can also cause conjunctival injection (vessel dilation).

Table 18.3 Red eye: differential diagnosis.

Deep red, sclera obscured	Subconjunctival haemorrhage
Diffuse bulbar and tarsal injection	Infective conjunctivitis
	Allergic conjunctivitis
	Angle closure glaucoma
	Reaction to topical medication
	Dry eyes
	In association with orbital cellulitis
Diffuse/focal bulbar injection	Episcleritis
	Scleritis
	Chemical injury
	Eyelid malposition
	Blepharitis
	Endophthalmitis
	Pingueculae
	Pterygia
Perilimbal (ciliary) injection	Iritis
	Keratitis
	Corneal abrasion
	Corneal ulcer
	Corneal foreign body

- *Chemical injury* may be associated with generalized or local conjunctival inflammation, but alkali burns may cause ischaemic whitening, signifying severe tissue damage.

Infection

The commonest site of infection is the conjunctiva itself.

- *Conjunctivitis* is a generalized inflammation of the conjunctiva associated with symptoms of discharge and mild discomfort rather than pain. Any visual blur due to discharge is cleared on blinking. Bacterial infections are associated with a purulent discharge that may stick the lids together. Viral infections cause a watery discharge and in severe cases, where the cornea is affected, the patient experiences photophobia and blurred vision. Chlamydial infections can produce a chronically red eye.
- *Malposition of the lids* (e.g. entropion) and *lid margin inflammation* (blepharitis) may cause secondary inflammation of the conjunctiva due to recurrent irritation. Blepharitis is usually without discharge and may be associated with acne rosacea, atopic dermatitis and other skin diseases. The patient complains of lid irritation or itching. In some cases, staphylococcal lid margin commensals may induce a

hypersensitivity (immune complex) reaction in the peripheral cornea resulting in a keratitis or marginal ulcer. This is accompanied by a ciliary injection.

• *Corneal infection* affecting the visual axis is sight-threatening and may be associated with localized or general ocular redness. The eye is painful, particularly in acanthamoeba keratitis, and the vision reduced. There may be a mucopurulent discharge. A background history of contact lens use is common as an initiating factor.

• *Intraocular infection* (endophthalmitis) may occasionally occur within days following intraocular surgery. It causes a marked generalized conjunctival inflammation. The eye is painful (unusual after routine intraocular surgery) and the vision reduced. A history of recent surgery is the clue. Such a patient requires immediate referral to an eye unit.

• An *infection of the orbit*, orbital cellulitis, presents with swollen and often erythematous lids. The conjunctiva may be swollen and red, and eye movements are reduced. The eye is proptosed. This is a medical emergency, for vision may be lost due to optic nerve damage

Acute glaucoma

The sudden rise in pressure associated with acute angle closure glaucoma, and other causes of acute glaucoma, result in a generalized red eye, corneal clouding, reduced vision and severe pain. It needs urgent treatment.

Other forms of inflammation

A number of other inflammatory diseases may present with a red eye, of which the commonest, mainly seen in primary care, is allergic eye disease.

• *Seasonal allergic conjunctivitis*, or hayfever conjunctivitis, is a common disorder, particularly in the spring and summer when exposure to allergens is at its height. The conjunctiva is injected and may be swollen (chemosed); the eye itches and waters and there is accompanying sneezing (due to allergic rhinitis) as part of the overall picture of hay fever. Vision is unaffected, but the eye may be photophobic. Vernal keratoconjunctivitis, a chronic form of allergic eye disease, will also present as a red irritable eye. There may be a history of atopy. With both there may be a mucus discharge.

• *Dry eyes* may also be associated with mild redness, irritation and 'tiredness' of the eye. In severe cases the vision may be blurred.

• In *episcleritis* the episcleral tissues are inflamed. This may result in focal or general inflammation, and may or may not be painful. There is no discharge, and the vision is not reduced.

• In *scleritis*, inflammation of the sclera is associated with the collagen vascular diseases. Again there may be focal or generalized inflammation of the sclera and overlying conjunctiva. The scleral inflammation is apparent, seen through the conjunctiva. Pain is deep and boring.

• Other conjunctival or corneal lesions, for example pterygia and pingueculae, may present with focal redness. The cause is usually easily visible.

• A red eye may be associated with topical medication, for example the prostaglandin analogues used in the treatment of glaucoma.

Sudden visual loss

Sudden uniocular loss of vision is caused either by a sudden clouding of the ocular media or by a problem with the retina or optic nerve. It is important to determine the onset and duration of the visual loss and whether there has been any progression or recovery. It is essential to establish that this is truly a *sudden* loss of vision and not simply a longstanding loss which has gone unnoticed, to be revealed when the fellow eye was covered. It is always important to identify any associated features, such as visual symptoms or pain (Table 18.4), which preceded visual loss.

A general medical history is vital. For example, is the patient diabetic or hypertensive?

Table 18.4 Sudden visual loss: causes.

Painful		Angle closure glaucoma
		Retrobulbar optic neuritis
		Giant cell arteritis
		Orbital cellulitis
		Uveitis
		Endophthalmitis
		Corneal ulcer/keratitis
Painless	Fleeting visual loss	Embolic arterial occlusion
		Migraine
		Raised intracranial pressure
		Prodromal in giant cell arteritis
	Prolonged visual loss	Ischaemic optic neuropathy
		Retinal artery occlusion
		Retinal vein occlusion
		Vitreous haemorrhage
		Retinal detachment
		Age-related macular degeneration
		Other macular disease
		Orbital disease affecting the optic nerve
		Intracranial disease affecting the visual pathway

Opacities of the transparent media of the eye

• The sudden onset of corneal oedema and clouding in *acute angle closure glaucoma* causes blurred vision, severe pain and redness of the eye. There may be a history of attacks of blurred vision and eye pain or headache which then subsided. Such prodromal attacks may be precipitated in the dark, by pupil dilation, which causes a subacute attack of angle closure glaucoma.

• Visual loss may also occur quite quickly with the development of a *corneal ulcer* or *keratitis*, again with redness, and usually but not always with severe pain.

• A *bleed into the vitreous* is a common cause of sudden, painless visual loss and may result from a rupture of abnormal fine capillary vessels growing from the surface of the retina (proliferative diabetic retinopathy) or associated with central retinal vein occlusion or 'wet' age-related macular degeneration. It may also be seen following a posterior vitreous detachment, when it may be associated with retinal hole formation and retinal detachment.

• *Anterior uveitis* may cause some blurring of vision when inflammatory cells adhering to the back of the cornea (keratic precipitates), or pupillary synechiae, lie on the visual axis.

• In *posterior uveitis*, visual loss may be caused by a vitritis (inflammation of the vitreous). This may be associated with a local retinitis or choroiditis, with further visual loss due to retinal damage. The eye will also be slightly painful and photophobic. *Endophthalmitis* is an extreme form of posterior uveitis, usually due to an intraocular bacterial infection following cataract surgery. It presents with a rapidly escalating painful and profound visual loss.

Retinal abnormalities

• *Total occlusion* of the central retinal vein or retinal artery results in a sudden painless loss of vision involving the whole visual field. A branch occlusion causes a partial loss of vision.

• Wet *age-related macular degeneration* can cause a sudden loss or distortion of vision. Central vision is lost but peripheral vision is retained. Other acute disorders affecting the macula, such as *central serous retinopathy* or a *macular hole*, may cause sudden central visual loss.

• A *retinal detachment* may be preceded by floaters, due either to a small vitreous bleed (see above) or to a vitreous detachment and condensation of the vitreous gel. Vitreous detachment also puts traction on the retina, giving rise to the key symptom of flashing lights. Detachment itself results in a curtain-like loss of the visual field, which starts at the top of the visual field in the case of an inferior detachment, or at the bottom of the field if the detachment is superior.

- Inflammation of the retina associated with a *posterior uveitis* may cause visual loss, particularly if the macula or optic nerve is involved.
- A transient loss of vision, lasting minutes and described as 'a shutter coming quickly across the vision', is typical of *amaurosis fugax*. It is caused by a platelet embolus passing through the retinal circulation.
- Occasionally, visual loss is attributable to a *migraine attack* causing vasospasm of the retinal vessels. More commonly migraine presents with fortification spectra or scintillating scotomata at the start of an attack.

Optic nerve abnormalities

- *Optic neuritis*, due to focal demyelination of the optic nerve, causes loss of vision which develops over a couple of days. With retrobulbar neuritis the optic nerve head appears normal and, when the optic sheath is involved, the patient complains of pain on eye movement. Anterior optic neuritis is accompanied by nerve head swelling, or papillitis.
- *Anterior ischaemic optic neuropathy* (AION) results from a sudden decrease in blood supply to the optic nerve head. It presents with loss of vision. It may be caused by *giant cell arteritis* (GCA), with associated symptoms of pain in the temple, jaw claudication, shoulder pain and tiredness. There is usually a profound loss of vision in the affected eye. GCA is a medical emergency requiring urgent treatment with steroids. AION may also be seen in patients with vascular disease accompanying ageing, diabetes or hypertension. The risk is increased in those with small, crowded optic discs. In these cases the loss of field is painless. Symptoms are often first noticed in the morning, perhaps reflecting the falls in blood pressure and optic nerve head perfusion pressure that occur during sleep. Visual loss commonly affects the upper or lower visual field.
- Episodes of visual loss lasting only a few seconds are typical of *raised intracranial pressure*. These visual 'obscurations' are often worse with a change in posture, and occur in the presence of papilloedema.
- The optic nerve may be compressed in orbital cellulitis, resulting in visual loss.

Visual loss involving both eyes

This usually suggests disease of the visual pathway including the optic nerves or visual cortices. Occasionally an ocular cause may be found, for example if both eyes are affected by uveitis.

Gradual visual loss

Patients may adjust to a gradual loss of vision, so there may be a lengthy delay

Table 18.5 Gradual visual loss: causes.

Media cloudy	
(opacities in the cornea, lens or vitreous appear black against the red reflex)	Corneal opacity
	Cataract
	Vitreous haemorrhage
Media clear	
Retinal disorder	Age-related macular degeneration
	Macular/retinal dystrophy
Optic nerve/pathway disorder	Optic neuropathy
	Central nervous disease affecting
	visual pathways (e.g. visual cortex)

before they seek medical help. This is particularly so in older patients with cataract. Also, in chronic glaucoma, because of its slow evolution, the patient may be unaware of a considerable degree of visual field loss until it is detected by chance or investigated when glaucoma is diagnosed at a routine assessment.

• Cloudy ocular media, due to the gradual development of corneal oedema, cataract or rarely vitreous opacity, are possible causes for a gradual, painless reduction in vision (Table 18.5).

• In patients with clear media, retinal abnormalities, particularly those affecting the macular region, may be present. Retinal dystrophies often cause a gradual reduction in vision. Dry macular degeneration may also result in a slow decline in central vision, sometimes accompanied by visual distortion.

• Compressive optic nerve disease is usually associated with gradual visual loss, which may also be caused by intracranial disease such as a pituitary tumour.

Ocular pain

The presence of pain can be very useful in deciding the cause of other ocular symptoms. It is seldom the only presenting feature of eye disease, and most causes have already been discussed. They are summarized in Table 18.6.

Diplopia

The onset of diplopia or double vision can be a worrying symptom, both for the patient and for the clinician! It is important, as ever, to obtain a full history (Table 18.7).

• The answers to these questions will often reveal the diagnosis. The most common cause of diplopia is a paresis due to disease of the third, fourth or sixth cranial nerve (Table 18.8). These are usually painless, constant and acute. Testing the eye

Table 18.6 Ocular pain: causes.

Discomfort	Blepharitis
	Dry eye
	Conjunctivitis
	Allergy
	Dysthyroid eye disease
Pain on eye movements	Optic neuritis
Pain around eye	Giant cell arteritis
	Migraine
	Orbital cellulitis
	Causes of 'headache'
Severe pain	Corneal abrasion / foreign body
	Keratitis
	Angle closure glaucoma
	Endophthalmitis
	Uveitis
	Scleritis
	Myositis

Table 18.7 Establishing the history in a patient with diplopia.

Was the onset sudden or gradual?
Is there a history of trauma?
Is the double vision present all the time?
Is it worse when the patient is tired?
Are the two images horizontally, vertically or diagonally (a skew deviation) displaced?
What are the associated symptoms (abnormalities of the pupils, other neurological symptoms)?
Are there any clues in the general medical history (diabetes, hypertension, thyroid disorders)?
Does the diplopia disappear when either eye is covered (to exclude a uniocular cause for the diplopia)?

movements reveals the type of palsy present. Inter- and supranuclear palsies may also present acutely. The nature of the disorder in eye movements usually helps locate the site of the lesion. Intermittent double vision is typical of myasthenia, where the symptoms are worse as the patient tires.

• If thyroid eye disease is suspected (Graves' disease), look for the other features of that condition as well as the characteristic restricted eye movements and acute inflammation over the insertion of the extraocular muscles.

Table 18.8 Diplopia: causes.

Neurogenic	III, IV, VI nerve palsies
	Inter- and supranuclear gaze palsies
	Failure to control a longstanding squint
	Associated with field defects (bitemporal hemianopia)
Myogenic	Thyroid eye disease
	Myasthenia
	Myositis
	Myopathy
Orbital	Trauma
	Space-occupying lesions
	Caroticocavernous sinus fistula
Monocular	Corneal disease
	Cataract

- Trauma may cause a neurogenic diplopia if the cranial nerves are damaged, and a restrictive diplopia if an orbital fracture has been caused, with trapping of orbital tissue, in the floor or medial wall of the orbit. Once again a good history will suggest the most likely diagnosis.
- Diplopia may result when a patient fails to control a longstanding squint. Here again the symptoms may be intermittent.
- Occasionally diplopia may have a monocular cause, usually corneal opacification or cataract. Cataract may cause a ghosting of vision rather than diplopia.

Key points

- The eye is part of the body and is often affected in systemic disease. Always seek associated features.
- A good ophthalmic history can initiate a differential diagnosis and influence subsequent clinical examination.

Multiple choice questions

1. Match the description with the most likely diagnosis. A patient presents with:

a A diffusely red, sticky eye; vision is unaffected.

b A red eye most marked at the limbus, with photophobia and blurred vision.

c Sudden onset of a local red patch on the sclera, associated with slight discomfort but with normal vision. The patient takes warfarin.

d A painful red eye and slightly blurred vision. They suffer from rheumatoid arthritis.

e A painful red eye, very blurred vision and discharge. There is a history of contact lens wear.

   i Corneal ulcer.

   ii Optic neuritis.

   iii Scleritis.

   iv Uveitis.

   v Allergic conjunctivitis.

   vi Subconjunctival haemorrhage.

   vii Episcleritis.

   viii Bacterial conjunctivitis.

   ix Corneal abrasion.

   x Corneal foreign body.

2. Match the description with the most likely diagnosis. A patient presents with:

a Floaters, flashes of light and a curtain-like loss of vision.

b Sudden loss of vision in one eye, jaw claudication and shoulder pain.

c A painful red eye, loss of vision, nausea.

d Loss of vision for seconds on standing from lying down.

e Loss of vision over a couple of days associated with pain on eye movement.

   i Optic neuritis.

   ii Retinal vein occlusion.

   iii Retinal artery occlusion.

   iv Retinal detachment.

   v Acute glaucoma.

   vi Vitreous haemorrhage.

   vii Orbital cellulitis.

   viii Raised intracranial pressure.

   ix Giant cell arteritis.

   x Endophthalmitis.

3. Match the description with the most likely diagnosis. A patient presents with:

a A watering eye present since birth, associated with intermittent stickiness but no redness of the conjunctiva.

b A watering eye in a 6-month-old child associated with a large cornea. The eye is not red.

c A watering eye in a 60-year-old man, associated with a lower lid that droops away from the eye.

d A sticky, watery, white eye in a 55-year-old woman.

e An acute, watery, red eye associated with photophobia in a 26-year-old man.

i Viral conjunctivitis.

ii Corneal ulcer.

iii Congenital nasolacrimal duct obstruction.

iv Acquired nasolacrimal duct obstruction.

v Corneal foreign body.

vi Congenital glaucoma.

vii Migraine.

viii Ectropion.

ix Entropion.

x Molluscum contagiosum.

4. Match the description with the most likely diagnosis. A patient presents with:

a Gradual loss of vision over some months, with increasing glare in the sun.

b Gradual loss of vision followed by more rapid loss, associated with distortion of central vision.

c Gradual loss of vision in the right eye, associated with a relative afferent pupillary defect.

d Gradual loss of vision in both eyes, with no relative afferent pupillary defect or media opacity.

e Gradually increasing blurring of vision some months following cataract surgery.

i Pituitary tumour.

ii Cortical infarct.

iii Corneal ulcer.

iv Cataract.

v Age-related macular degeneration.

vi Macular oedema.

vii Optic nerve compression.

viii Retinal detachment.

ix Posterior capsule opacification.

5. Name the major sign in each of the photographs (Fig. 18.1).

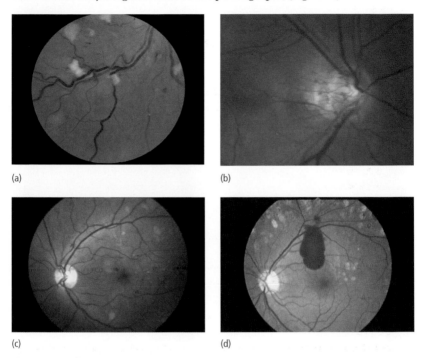

(a)

(b)

(c)

(d)

Figure 18.1 See Question 5.

6. Name the sign or condition in each case (Fig. 18.2).

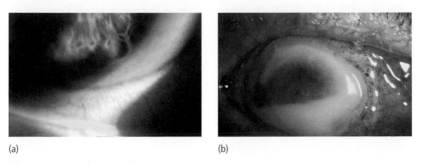

(a)

(b)

Figure 18.2 See Question 6.

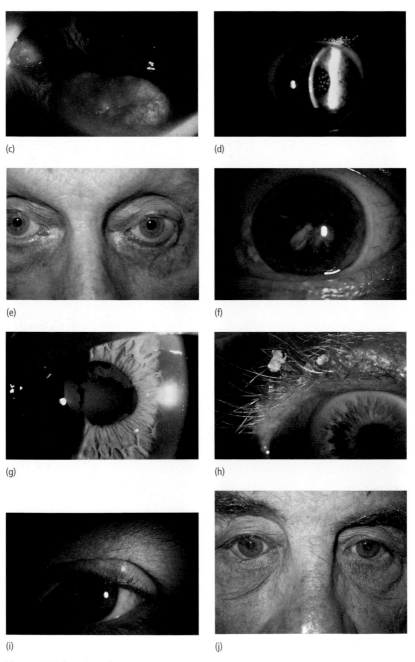

(c)

(d)

(e)

(f)

(g)

(h)

(i)

(j)

Figure 18.2 (*continued*)

7. What does this pathological section show (Fig. 18.3)? What is the diagnosis?

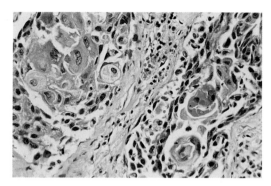

Figure 18.3 See Question 7.

8. What does this X-ray show (Fig. 18.4)? What is the diagnosis? How might the eyes be affected?

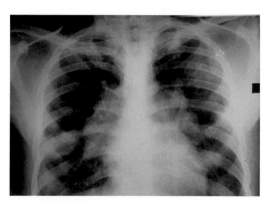

Figure 18.4 See Question 8.

Answers

1. Match the description with the diagnosis.

a Bacterial conjunctivitis.

b Uveitis.

c Subconjunctival haemorrhage.

d Scleritis.

e Corneal ulcer.

2. Match the description with the diagnosis.

a Retinal detachment.

b Giant cell arteritis.

c Acute glaucoma.

d Raised intracranial pressure.

e Optic neuritis.

3. Match the description with the diagnosis.

a Congenital nasolacrimal duct obstruction.

b Congenital glaucoma.

c Ectropion.

d Acquired nasolacrimal duct obstruction.

e Viral conjunctivitis.

4. Match the description with the diagnosis.

a Cataract.

b Age-related macular degeneration.

c Optic nerve compression.

d Pituitary tumour.

e Posterior capsule opacification.

5. Name the sign(s) in each of the photographs (Fig. 18.1).

a Cotton-wool spots, a few haemorrhages and escudates.

b Disc new vessels.

c Exudates, haemorrhages and cotton-wool spots.

d Pre-retinal haemorrhage, laser burns.

6. Name the sign or condition in each case (Fig. 18.2).

a Hyphaema.

b Hypopyon.

c Follicles.

d Keratitic precipitates.

e Ectropion.

f Cataract.

g Posterior synechiae.

h Anterior blepharitis.

i Meibomian cyst.

j Entropion.

7. What does this pathological section show (Fig. 18.3)?

• The slide shows giant cells seen in giant cell or temporal arteritis.

8. What does this X-ray show (Fig. 18.4)?

• The X-ray shows hilar lymphadenopathy seen in sarcoidosis; this may cause uveitis.

Chapter 19

Services for the visually handicapped

Learning objectives

To understand:
- The social help available to blind people.
- The reasons for registering a patient in the UK.

Introduction

Blindness has not been satisfactorily defined. Legally it is said to be 'so blind as to be unable to perform any work for which sight is essential'. This definition is none too helpful and each case must be assessed on its individual merits. The effects of reduced vision are influenced by:
- The speed and age at which it occurred (sudden visual loss is harder to adjust to than a gradual loss; younger people may be able to adapt better to poor vision than older people).
- Whether central or peripheral vision is affected.
- The type of field defect that is present. Homonymous hemianopia may present special difficulties in reading and navigation.
- The existence of other disabilities (e.g. deafness).

Help and advice are available in the UK both from local government (social services) and from voluntary organizations such as the Royal National Institute of the Blind (RNIB). There are also numerous local groups that offer support. Help is aimed at enabling the visually impaired person to lead an independent life.

Blind registration

In the UK, patients with poor vision who meet certain requirements can be registered as either partially sighted or blind, depending on the level of visual deficit. Blind registration does not necessarily mean that the person can see nothing at all. This helps to coordinate the services available for the patient. Not all patients wish to be registered, however, because of an assumed stigma, and it is important to discuss the subject fully with the patient. Despite the benefits that may follow registration, some patients regard it as an end to a fight against failing sight rather than a new beginning, managing the problem with all available help. It is important not to dismiss the wishes of these patients in trying to maximize their ability to manage their reduced vision. Registration is performed by an ophthalmologist. The benefits of registration, some only available to patients registered blind, include:

• Financial help (e.g. increased tax allowances, additional income support, disability living allowance, attendance allowance).
• Help from the social services (e.g. specialist assessment, adaptation of living accommodation).
• Exemption from directory enquiry fees.
• Public transport travel concessions, railcards, disabled parking schemes for carers.
• Help with access to work.

Patients with impaired sight, whether registered or not, may also benefit from the 'talking book and newspaper' schemes, which provide extensive recorded material. Further information is available from the RNIB website (www.rnib.org.uk).

Services for children with impaired sight

Children with impaired sight may require additional help with education, or may be educated in special schools for the visually handicapped. The local education authority has to make a *statement* of the educational needs of the child. Special visual aids, including voice-activated computers and closed-circuit television, may help.

In addition, children may be eligible for the disability living allowance, which may enable parents to claim additional benefits.

Additional help

As well as low-vision aids (see Chapter 3), various devices are available, ranging from telephones with large number buttons, and guides that help with placing a signature on a cheque, to devices that indicate when a cup is filled. Additionally, for some patients, training in the use of a cane or guide dog may aid mobility. Some patients may also benefit from learning Braille.

Key points

- Ensure that the patient is helped to maximize residual vision.
- Ensure that the patient is aware of support services, and if appropriate has been registered partially sighted or blind.
- Ensure that appropriate steps are taken for the education of a poorly sighted child.

Chapter 20

Clinical cases

Introduction

These case histories are designed to test your understanding of the symptoms, signs and management of ophthalmic disease that have been discussed in this book. Answers are given after each case and include references to chapters where additional information may be found.

Clinical cases

Case 1

A 70-year-old woman presents to the eye casualty department with sudden loss of vision in her right eye. She has noted increasing headache and her scalp is tender when she combs her hair. She complains of pain in the jaw when she eats, and tires easily. There is no ophthalmic history but she suffers from peptic ulceration. She takes no regular medications. There is no family history of medical problems.

Examination reveals a visual acuity of counting fingers in the affected eye. A relative afferent pupillary defect is present (see Chapter 2). The optic disc appears slightly swollen (Fig. 20.1). The left eye is normal.

Questions
- What is the likely diagnosis?
- What is the immediate treatment?
- How would you confirm the diagnosis?
- What other precautions would you take?

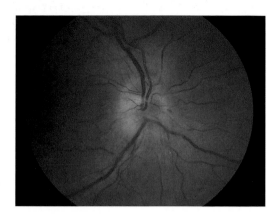

Figure 20.1 The appearance of the optic disc in case 1.

Answers

The patient almost certainly has giant cell arteritis causing ischaemic optic neuropathy (see Chapter 14). Intravenous and oral steroids must be given *immediately* before any other diagnostic step is taken, for there is a risk of arteritis and blindness in the fellow eye.

An ESR, CRP and temporal artery biopsy would help to confirm the diagnosis.

As the patient is being treated with steroids it is important to check a chest X-ray to exclude TB (steroids may cause miliary TB to develop if the disease is present). Blood pressure and blood glucose must be monitored. The patient should be warned of the other complications of steroid therapy, including immunosuppressive effects. Treatment to prevent osteoporosis is required. A positive history of gastric ulceration indicates that prophylactic treatment with a proton pump inhibitor will be required.

Case 2

A 40-year-old man presents with sudden onset of a drooping left eyelid. When he lifts the lid with his finger he notices that he has double vision. He has a severe headache. He is otherwise fit and well with no past ophthalmic history. He is on no regular medication. There is no family history of medical problems.

Examination reveals normal visual acuity in both eyes. A left ptosis is present. The left pupil is dilated. The left eye is abducted in the primary position of gaze. Testing of eye movements reveals reduced adduction elevation, and depression of the left eye. The remainder of the eye examination is normal.

Questions

- What nerve palsy is present?
- What is the most likely cause?
- What is the management?

Answers

The man has a third nerve palsy (see Chapter 15). An aneurysm from the posterior communicating artery pressing on the third nerve must be the initial diagnosis in a painful third nerve palsy. The patient requires urgent neurosurgical investigation with a magnetic resonance angiogram (MRA) and possibly angiography. Urgent treatment may be required. It is also important to check blood pressure and blood glucose. Diabetics may develop a painful third nerve palsy, but the pupil is not always affected (a "pupil-sparing third nerve palsy").

Case 3

A 55-year-old man presents to his GP with a five-day history of sudden onset of floaters in the left eye. These were accompanied by small flashes of light. He has treated hypertension but no other medical problems.

The GP examines the eye and finds a normal visual acuity. Dilated fundoscopy reveals no abnormality.

Questions

- What should the GP advise?
- What is the diagnosis?
- What are the associated risks?

Answers

As the symptoms are acute the GP should arrange for an urgent ophthalmic assessment. The man has a posterior vitreous detachment. The flashing lights are caused by traction of the vitreous gel on the retina. A specialized examination of the peripheral retina is needed. A tear may occur in the retina, which in turn may lead to a retinal detachment. Laser applied around the tear while it is flat can prevent retinal detachment (see Chapter 11).

Case 4

A 75-year-old woman attends the main casualty department with nausea and vomiting. She says that her right eye is painful and red. Vision is reduced. She wears glasses for near and distance vision. She is generally fit. There is no family history of medical problems.

On examination the casualty officer finds the vision to be reduced to counting fingers. The eye is red, the cornea appears cloudy and oedematous, and the pupil is oval and dilated on the affected side. No view of the fundus is obtained.

Questions
- What is the diagnosis?
- How might it be confirmed?
- What is the treatment?

Answers
The lady has acute angle closure glaucoma (see Chapter 10). Tonometry would reveal a high intraocular pressure (see Chapter 2). Gonioscopy would confirm the presence of a closed angle and a narrow angle in the fellow eye (see Chapter 10). The pressure must be lowered with intravenous acetazolamide and topical hypotensive drops including pilocarpine to produce miosis. A peripheral iridotomy is then performed, usually with a YAG laser in both eyes, to prevent further attacks.

Case 5

A 28-year-old man presents to his optician with a painful, red right eye. The vision has become increasingly blurred over the last two days. He wears soft contact lenses, and contact lens tolerance has decreased in the preceding days.

The optician notes that the vision is reduced to 6/60 in the right eye, the conjunctiva is inflamed, and there is a central opacity on the cornea. A small hypopyon (see Chapter 9) is present (Fig. 20.2).

Questions
- What is the likely diagnosis?
- What should the optician do?

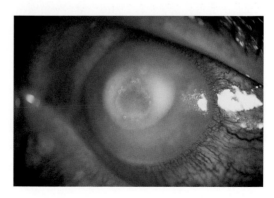

Figure 20.2 The appearance of the eye in case 5.

Answers
It is likely that the man has an infective corneal ulcer. He requires immediate referral to an ophthalmic casualty unit. The ulcer will be scraped for culture and the contact lens and any containers cultured. Intensive, topical, broad-spectrum antibiotics are administered as an inpatient pending the result of the microbiological investigation (see Chapter 7).

Case 6

A mother attends her GP's surgery with her baby, now 8 months old. He has had a persistently watery eye since birth. Intermittently there is a yellow discharge surrounding the eye. The white of the eye has never been red. The baby is otherwise healthy.

Examination reveals a white, quiet, normal eye. Slight pressure over the lacrimal sac produces a yellowish discharge from the normal puncta.

Questions
- What is the diagnosis?
- What advice would you give the mother?

Answers
It is likely that the child has an imperforate nasolacrimal duct. The mother should be reassured that this often resolves spontaneously. The lids should be kept clean and the skin over the lacrimal sac massaged gently on a daily basis. Antibiotics are generally not effective. If the symptoms persist after the child's first birthday the child can be referred to an ophthalmologist for syringing and probing of the nasolacrimal duct (see Chapter 6).

Case 7

A 14-year-old complains of intermittent redness and soreness of the right eye. He has noticed a small lump on the upper lid. The vision is unaffected.

Examination reveals a small raised lesion on the skin of the upper lid, associated with a follicular conjunctivitis below (Fig. 20.3).

Questions
- What is the likely diagnosis?
- What is the treatment?

Answers
It is likely that the lid lesion is a molluscum contagiosum. It is treated by excision (see Chapter 5).

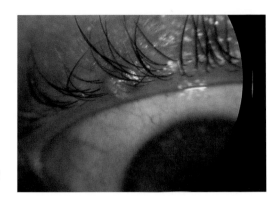

Figure 20.3 The appearance of the lid in case 7.

Case 8

A 35-year-old man presents to his GP with erythematous, swollen right upper and lower eyelids, worsening over the previous two days. He is unable to open them. He feels unwell and has a temperature.

Examination reveals marked lid swelling, a tender globe and, on manual opening of the lids, a proptosis with chemotic injected conjunctiva. Eye movements are limited in all directions. Visual acuity and colour vision are normal, and there is no relative afferent pupillary defect (see Chapter 2). The optic disc and retina also appear normal.

Questions
- What is the diagnosis?
- What is the management?

Answers
The man has orbital cellulitis (see Chapter 4). Blood cultures and a high nasal swab should be performed, together with an orbital CT scan, to confirm the diagnosis and delineate any abscess. He requires admission to hospital for intravenous antibiotics and close monitoring of his vision, colour vision and pupillary reflexes, as he is at risk of severe optic nerve damage. The ENT surgeons should be informed, as they may be required to drain an abscess. The normal acuity and colour vision suggest that the optic nerve is not compromised at present, but should these change for the worse urgent surgical drainage will be required.

Case 9

While working in the laboratory a colleague inadvertently sprays his eyes with an alkali solution.

Questions
- What is the immediate treatment?
- What should you do next?

Answers
The eyes must be washed out with copious quantities (litres) of water immediately. Alkalis are very toxic to the eye. Failure to treat immediately may result in permanent, severe ocular damage (see Chapter 16). The patient should then be taken to an eye emergency clinic.

Case 10

A 27-year-old man presents with a two-day history of a painful red right eye; the vision is slightly blurred and he dislikes bright lights. He is otherwise fit and well, but complains of some backache. He wears no glasses.

Questions
- What is the likely diagnosis?
- What would you expect to find on examination of the eye?
- What treatment would you give?
- What is the eye condition likely to be associated with?

Answers
The patient has iritis (see Chapter 9). Examination would reveal a reduction in visual acuity, redness of the eye that is worse at the limbus, cells in the anterior chamber and possibly on the cornea (keratic precipitate) or a collection at the bottom of the anterior chamber (hypopyon). The iris may be stuck to the lens (posterior synechiae). There may be inflammation of the vitreous and retina. The patient is treated with steroid eye drops to reduce the inflammation and dilating drops to prevent the formation of posterior synechiae. The history of backache suggests that the patient may have ankylosing spondylitis.

Case 11

A 68-year-old lady presents with a mildly painful red eye and some blurring of vision. One year previously she had a corneal graft. She is on no medications and is otherwise well.

Questions
- What is the possible diagnosis?
- What treatment should the patient be given?

Answers

There may be a number of causes of this lady's red eye. A diagnosis of graft rejection must be considered first of all. The patient must be referred to an eye department as an emergency. If a graft rejection is confirmed, she will need intensive treatment with topical steroids to save the graft (see Chapter 7).

Case 12

A 68-year-old hypertensive man noted a fleeting loss of vision in one eye lasting for about a minute. He described it as a curtain coming down over the vision. Recovery was complete. There was no pain.

Examination reveals no abnormality.

Questions
- What is the diagnosis?
- What treatment would you advise?

Answers

The patient has had an episode of amaurosis fugax, most likely caused by the passage of a fibrin-platelet embolus through the retinal arteriolar circulation. The patient requires treatment with antiplatelet drugs and a cardiovascular work-up. The most likely abnormality is a plaque on the carotid artery, which may require surgery (see Chapter 12).

Case 13

A 60-year-old lady presented to her GP with gradual loss of vision over some months. She noticed that the problem was particularly bad in bright sunshine. The eye was not painful or red. She was otherwise well.

Questions
- What is the probable diagnosis?
- How can the diagnosis be confirmed?
- What treatment may be advised?

Answers

It is likely that the lady has a cataract. These can be readily seen with a slit lamp, but are also well visualized with the direct ophthalmoscope in the red reflex (Fig. 20.4). The advantages and possible complications of cataract surgery should be discussed with her once the diagnosis has been confirmed (see Chapter 8).

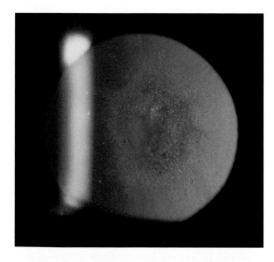

Figure 20.4 The red reflex seen with direct ophthalmoscopy in case 13.

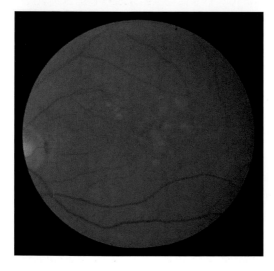

Figure 20.5 The appearance of the macula in case 14.

Case 14

An 80-year-old lady who has already lost the vision in one eye develops distortion and reduction of vision over a few days in her good eye.

Examination reveals an acuity of 6/12, an early cataract and an abnormality at the macula (Fig. 20.5).

Questions
- What is the likely diagnosis?
- What treatment may be helpful?

Answers
The rapid onset suggests that the cataract has little to do with the new visual disturbance. It is most likely due to age-related macular degeneration (AMD) (see Chapter 11). In some patients, following a fluorescein angiogram, laser therapy or anti-VEGF injections may be helpful in preventing further progression.

Case 15

A 30-year-old builder was using a hammer to hit a steel chisel. He felt something hit his eye and the vision became blurred. He is fit and well and there is no history of medical problems.

On examination by his GP the vision was reduced to 6/12. A fluorescein-staining lesion was seen on the cornea but this appeared Seidel's-negative. A small hyphaema was seen in the anterior chamber, and in the red reflex observed with a direct ophthalmoscope a well-delineated lens opacity was seen. The retina appeared normal.

Questions
- What is the cause of the reduced acuity?
- What is the likely origin of the lens opacity?
- What is the possible management of the patient?

Answers
It is likely that a piece of steel travelling at high velocity has penetrated the cornea, caused damage to the iris (resulting in the hyphaema) and passed into or through the lens (causing the opacity). The relatively good acuity suggests that there has been no damage to the macular region of the retina. The patient needs to be seen urgently in an eye unit. The corneal wound, if self-sealing, will probably not require suturing. The exact location of the foreign body has to be determined. Although it is unlikely to cause an infection (heat generated by the impact of the hammer on the metal may effectively sterilize the fragment) it may cause retinal toxicity if it has entered the vitreous cavity or retina. If it is enclosed in the lens (Fig. 20.6) there is less chance of retinal toxicity developing but the patient is at high risk of developing a subsequent cataract that may require operation. A foreign body that impacts on the retina or the vitreous body requires a vitrectomy to remove it, with careful examination of the retina for tears (see Chapter 16).

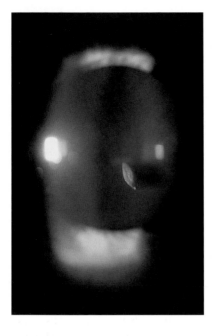

Figure 20.6 The intralenticular foreign body seen in case 15.

Case 16

A 2-year-old child was thought to have a squint by her parents. The finding was confirmed by her GP and she was referred to hospital.

Question
• What examination must be conducted in hospital?

Answer
Having taken a full history, an orthoptist will measure the visual acuity of the child, examine the range of eye movements, determine the presence type of squint with a cover test, trying to assess the degree of binocular vision present. The child will have a refraction performed and glasses prescribed if there is a significant refractive error or a difference in the strength of the lens needed between the two eyes (anisometropia). An ophthalmologist will examine the eye to check that there is no ocular or neurological condition that may account for the squint (see Chapter 15).

Case 17

A 26-year-old lady presents with a three-day history of blurring of vision in the right eye. This has become progressively worse. She also has pain caused by moving the eye. She has previously had an episode of weakness in the right arm two years ago, but this settled without treatment. She is otherwise fit and well.

On examination in ophthalmic casualty the vision was recorded as 6/60, with no improvement on looking through a pinhole. The eye was white and quiet with no abnormality noted save for a right relative afferent pupillary defect (see Chapter 2).

Questions
- What is the diagnosis?
- How could this be confirmed?
- What are the management options?
- What is the prognosis?

Answers
The patient has the typical symptoms and signs of optic neuritis (see Chapter 14). The diagnosis can be supported by an MRI scan to look for additional plaques of demyelination and a visual evoked potential to examine the functioning of the optic nerve. A neurologist may also suggest performing a lumbar puncture, particularly if there is any doubt about the diagnosis. With the possibility of a previous neurological episode it is likely that the patient has multiple sclerosis. It is of great importance that appropriate counselling is given. Steroid treatment may speed up the recovery of vision and the prognosis for recovery of vision over a few months is good.

Case 18

A 79-year-old man presents with a lesion on his right lower lid (Fig. 20.7). It has been there for some months and has gradually grown bigger. It is ulcerated and the ulcer shows a pearly margin.

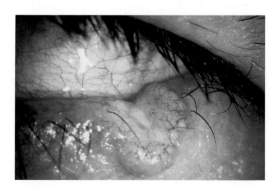

Figure 20.7 The appearance of the lid in case 18.

Questions
- What is the lesion?
- How should it be treated?

Answers
This is a basal cell carcinoma. It requires local excision. There is no problem with metastatic spread but local extension could cause severe problems as the tumour grows and infiltrates surrounding structures (see Chapter 5).

Case 19

A 60-year-old man presents with tired sore eyes. He has noted that the eyelids may crust in the morning. Sometimes the white of the eye is red. The vision is unaffected. He is otherwise fit and well.

Questions
- What is the probable diagnosis?
- What signs would you look for?
- How can this condition be treated?

Answers
The patient has blepharitis (see Chapter 5). Scaling of the lid margins and at the base of the lashes, together with inflammation of the lid margins and plugging of the meibomian glands, may be present (Fig. 20.8). Lid cleaning, along with the use of local antibiotic ointment and possibly topical steroids (supervised by an ophthalmologist), will improve, if not alleviate, the symptoms. Heat and lid massage can restore oil flow. If associated with acne rosacea, systemic tetracycline treatment may be beneficial.

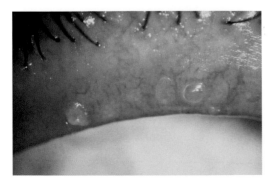

Figure 20.8 Plugging of the meibomian glands in case 19.

Case 20

A 30-year-old man develops an acute red eye associated with a watery discharge. Vision is unaffected but the eye irritates. He is otherwise fit and well.

Questions
- What is the diagnosis?
- What confirmatory signs would you look for on examination?
- What precautions would you take following your examination?

Answers
The patient has viral conjunctivitis (see Chapter 7). Examination for a preauricular lymph node and conjunctival follicles on the lower tarsus would confirm the diagnosis. This form of conjunctivitis is highly contagious; it is important to ensure that hands and equipment are thoroughly cleaned following the examination, and that the importance of good hygiene is emphasized to the patient.

Chapter 21

Useful references

Textbooks

Listed below are some sources that will provide more detailed information about the subjects covered in this book.

Clinical ophthalmology

American Academy of Ophthalmology. Basic and Clinical Science Course (BCSC), 2006–2007. (Reviews of ophthalmic subspecialty subjects.)

Easty, D. L. & Sparrow, J. M. (eds) (1999) *Oxford Textbook of Ophthalmology*. Oxford University Press. (Large comprehensive textbook from Britain.)

Kanski, J. J. (2003) *Clinical Ophthalmology*. Fifth edition. Butterworth-Heinemann. (Concise illustrated description of ophthalmic disease.)

Kanski, J. J. (2002) *Clinical Ophthalmology: a Test Yourself Atlas*. Butterworth-Heinemann. (Test your knowledge with this companion volume.)

Kunimoto, D. Y., Kanitkar, K. D. & Makar, M. (eds) (2004) *The Wills Eye Manual*. Fourth edition. Lippincott, Williams & Wilkins. (Concise details on the management of ophthalmic disease.)

Rowe, F. J. (2004) *Clinical Orthoptics*. Second edition. Blackwell Science. (Outlines the examination and diagnosis of eye movement disorders.)

Spalton, D. J., Hitchings, R. A. & Hunter, P. A. (2005) *Atlas of Clinical Ophthalmology*. Third edition. Mosby. (Illustrated account of ophthalmic disease.)

Yanoff, M., Duker, J. S. & Augsburger, J. J. (eds) (2003) *Ophthalmology*. Second edition. Mosby. (Also available on CD-ROM.) (Large comprehensive textbook from America.)

Basic science

Bron, A. J., Tripathi, R. C. & Tripathi, B. J. (1997) *Wolff's Anatomy of the Eye and Orbit*. Eighth edition. Chapman & Hall.

Elkington, A. R. (1999) *Clinical Optics*. Third edition. Blackwell Science.

Forrester, J. V. *et al.* (2001) *The Eye: Basic Sciences in Practice*. Second edition. Saunders.

Snell, R. S. & Lemp, M. A. (1998) *Clinical Anatomy of the Eye*. Second edition. Blackwell Science.

Review journals

Eye News

Published by Pinpoint Ltd. Provides short practical review articles and information about new developments in ophthalmology.

Survey of Ophthalmology

Published by Elsevier Science. Bi-monthly. Provides in-depth well-referenced review articles on particular topics in ophthalmology.

Ophthalmic journals

For detailed research articles there are numerous ophthalmic publications; most of the subspecialty fields in ophthalmology have their own journal. Among the leaders in clinical ophthalmology are:

American Journal of Ophthalmology

Archives of Ophthalmology

British Journal of Ophthalmology

Eye

Experimental Eye Research

Graefe's Archive for Clinical and Experimental Ophthalmology

Ophthalmology

Investigative Ophthalmology and Visual Science (IOVS)

Websites

www.rcophth.ac.uk. The Royal College of Ophthalmologists. Includes details of the college's publications and information about ophthalmic disease for patients.

www.aao.org. The American Academy of Ophthalmology. Test your knowledge of basic science. Contains updates on every aspect of ophthalmology.

www.djo.harvard.edu. The Digital Journal of Ophthalmology. Includes clinical case presentations and quizzes from the large American ophthalmic hospitals.

www.icoph.org. The International Council of Ophthalmology. Includes a comprehensive list of ophthalmic journals with links to their websites. Information about educational meetings. Information about eye diseases for patients linking to other websites.

www.eyecasualty.co.uk. The Oxford Eye Hospital. This provides details on common ocular emergencies, and patient information sheets on common eye problems.

www.mrcophth.com. Information about training hospitals in the UK, the addresses of the surgical colleges, a link to the BMJ ophthalmology job pages and a discussion board for those in training.

www.moorfields.nhs.uk. The Moorfields Eye Hospital. Describes the facilities of the hospital, courses available, and has information sheets for patients on common eye diseases.

www.rnib.org.uk. The Royal National Institute of the Blind. Produces a range of fact sheets for patients.

www.ophthalmologyresources.com. Sponsored by a large pharmaceutical company, the website is aimed at ophthalmologists but will help students seeking more detailed information about ophthalmic topics.

www.optometry.co.uk. Website of *Optometry Today*, the journal of the Association of Optometrists. It is accessed online and contains clinical review articles.

www.pinpointmedical.com/eye_news/eye_home.html. The *Eye News* website contains a directory of companies involved in the manufacture of ophthalmic equipment and medicines. Some of these sites also contain clinical information.

www.glaucoma-association.com. The International Glaucoma Association provides patient-orientated information about glaucoma.

www.maculardisease.org. The website of the Macular Disease Society provides patient-orientated information about macular disease.

www.lshtm.ac.uk. The London School of Hygiene and Tropical Medicine website, for those wishing to find out more about tropical ophthalmology.

www.v2020.org. Vision 2020: this site describes the activities of the programme to eliminate preventable world blindness by 2020.

Organizations producing patient information literature

The Royal National Institute of the Blind, 105 Judd Street, London WC1H 9NE, UK. Produces a variety of leaflets on common ocular conditions from the patient's perspective. It is also a most valuable source of information and practical help for visually impaired people.

The Royal College of Ophthalmologists, 17 Cornwall Terrace, London NW1 4QW, UK.

American Academy of Ophthalmology, PO Box 7424, San Francisco, CA 94120-7424, USA. Produces a range of booklets and guidelines on ophthalmic topics.

Appendix

Visual acuity equivalence table

United States notation (feet)	Metres	Expressed as a decimal
20/200	6/60	1.0
20/160	6/48	0.9
20/125	6/37	0.8
20/100	6/30	0.7
20/80	6/24	0.6
20/60	6/18	0.5
20/50	6/15	0.4
20/40	6/12	0.3
20/30	6/9	0.2
20/25	6/7	0.1
20/20	6/6	0.0
20/16	6/5	−0.1
20/12.5	6/3.8	−0.2
20/10	6/3	−0.3

The following abbreviations are also used

CF   Count Fingers. The ability to count fingers at a specified distance.

HM   Hand Movements. The ability to see a hand moving in front of the face.

LP   Light Perception. The ability to differentiate light from dark.

NLP   No Light Perception. Unable to detect light.

Index

Page numbers in *italics* represent figures, those in **bold** represent tables.

Index

Index

posterior chamber 2, 2
preferential looking test 25
presbyopia 46, 47
preseptal cellulitis 53, 55
proptosis 39, 51–2, 52, 74, 219, 219
pseudoexfoliative glaucoma 131
Pseudomonas spp. 89
pseudopapilloedema 195
pseudophakia 47
psoriasis 115
pterygium 86, 86, 259
ptosis 4, 33, 60–2, 61
  management 62
  pathogenesis 61
  signs 62
  symptoms 61
puncta 4, 5
punctate staining 73
pupil 12, 185–91
  Adie's 188
  Argyll Robertson 188
  drugs affecting **189**
pupillary abnormality
  light-near dissociation 187–9
    Adie's pupil 188
    Argyll Robertson pupil 188
    midbrain pupil 188
    relative afferent pupillary defect 187–8
  neurological causes 186–7, 187
  ocular causes 186
pupillary control pathway 186
pupillary reactions 30, 32, 32
pursuit movements 33

quandritic defects 28

radiological imaging 40
raised intracranial pressure **195**, 196–7, 261
recurrent corneal erosion syndrome 235, 238
red eye 255–6, **256**, **257**
  differential diagnosis **257**
  see also conjunctivitis
refractive error 214
refractive surgery 48–9
Reiter's disease 115, 119
relative afferent pupillary defect 32, 187–8
retina 2, 7, 8, 11, 14, 145
  acquired macular disease 146–53
    age-related macular degeneration 147–9, 148, 260
    central serous retinopathy 151, 151

macular holes and membranes 150, 150
    macular oedema 151, 152
    toxic maculopathies 152, 153
  albinism 161
  anatomical examination 35–7, 36, 37
  dialysis 229, 234, 237
  inherited and photoreceptor dystrophies 158–60
    cone dystrophy 160
    retinitis pigmentosa 158–60, 159
    juvenile macular dystrophies 160
    macular dysfunction 146
    peripheral retinal dysfunction 146
    posterior vitreous detachment 153–4, 153
    vitreous floaters 153–4, 153
retinal blood vessel abnormalities 181
retinal detachment 108, 154–8, 260, 276
  bullous 155
  retinoschisis 158
  rhegmatogenous 154–8, 155–8
  tractional 158
retinal pigment epithelium 7, 8–9, 8, 14
retinal tumours 161–3
retinal vascular disease 169–84
  abnormal retinal blood vessels 181
  arterial occlusion 176–7, 176
  arteriosclerosis and hypertension 179
  blood abnormalities 181
  diabetic retinopathy 171–6, **173**, 174, 175
  retinopathy of prematurity 179–80, 180
  sickle cell retinopathy 181
  signs of 169–71, 170
    vascular leakage 169, 171
    vascular occlusion 171
  venous occlusion 177–9, 178
retinitis 115
retinitis pigmentosa 24, 158–60, 159
retinoblastoma 161–3, 162
retinochoroiditis 121
retinopathy of prematurity 179–80
retinoschisis 158
retinoscopy 38
rhabdomyosarcoma 54, 57
rhegmatogenous retinal detachment 154–8, 155–8
  epidemiology 154–5, 155
  management 156–8, 157
  prognosis 158
  signs 155–6, 156
  symptoms 155
rods 7, 9, 10
Roth spots 181, 182
rubeosis iridis 131, 131